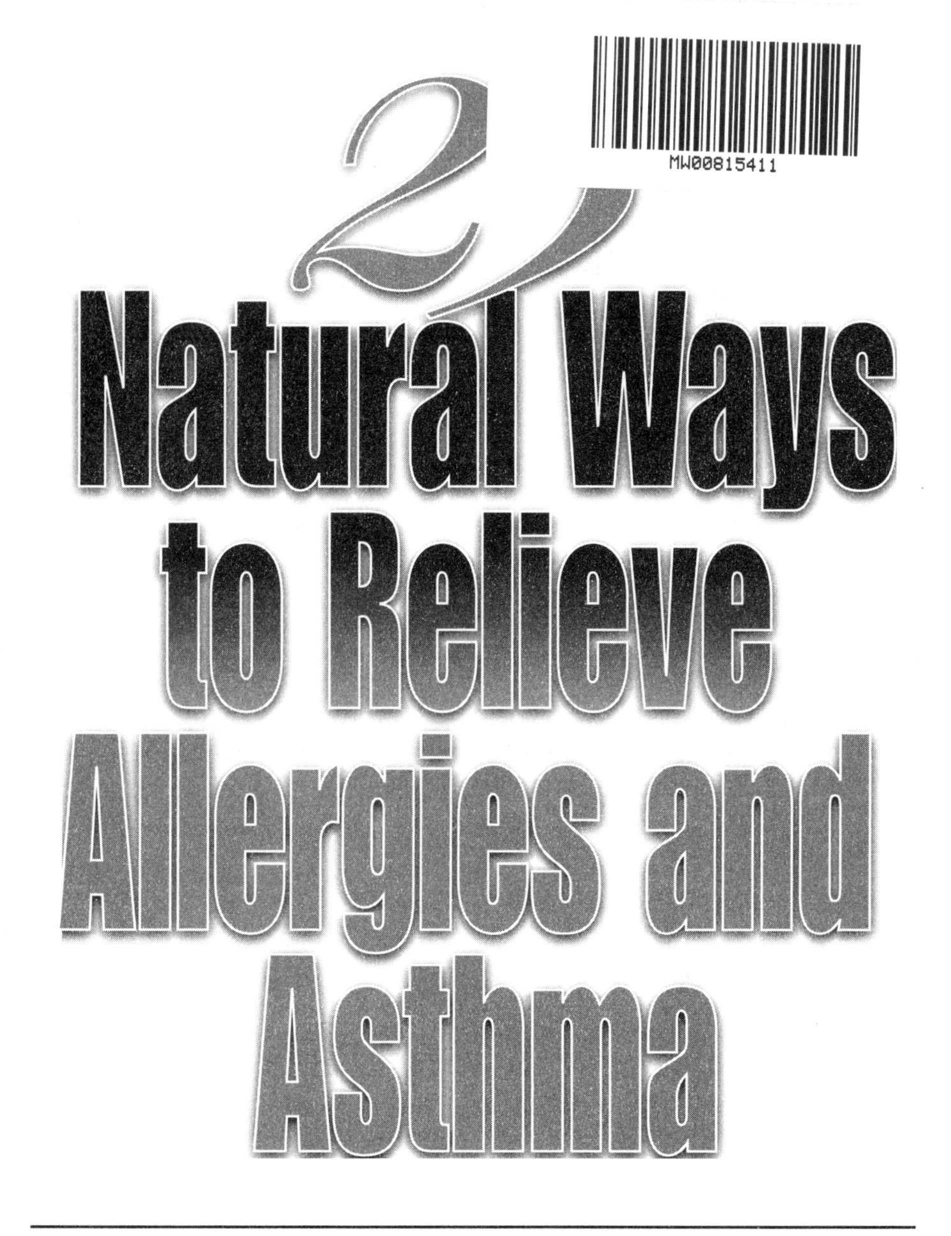

ROMY FOX

Keats Publishing

Chicago New York San Francisco Lisbon London Madrid Mexico City Milan New Delhi San Juan Seoul Singapore Sydney Toronto

Library of Congress Cataloging-in-Publication Data

Fox, Romy.
25 natural ways to relieve allergies and asthma : a mind-body approach to health and well-being / Romy Fox.
p. cm. — (25 natural ways . . . series)
Includes index.
ISBN 0-658-01374-2
1. Allergy—Alternative treatment. 2. Asthma—Alternative treatment. 3. Naturopathy. 4. Mind and body. I. Title: Twenty-five natural ways to relieve allergies and asthma. II. Title. III. Series.

RC585 .F685 2001

2001038132

Keats Publishing

A Division of The **McGraw·Hill** *Companies*

1 2 3 4 5 6 7 8 9 0 DOC/DOC 0 9 8 7 6 5 4 3 2 1

ISBN 0-658-01374-2

This book was set in Adobe Garamond
Printed and bound by R. R. Donnelley—Crawfordsville

Cover and series design by Wendy Staroba Loreen

McGraw-Hill books are available at special quantity discounts to use as premiums and sales promotions, or for use in corporate training programs. For more information, please write to the Director of Special Sales, Professional Publishing, McGraw-Hill, Two Penn Plaza, New York, NY 10121-2298. Or contact your local bookstore.

The purpose of this book is to educate. It is sold with the understanding that the publisher and author shall have neither liability nor responsibility for any injury caused or alleged to be caused directly or indirectly by the information contained in this book. While every effort has been made to ensure its accuracy, the book's contents should not be construed as medical advice. Each person's health needs are unique. To obtain recommendations appropriate to your particular situation, please consult a qualified health care provider.

This book is printed on acid-free paper.

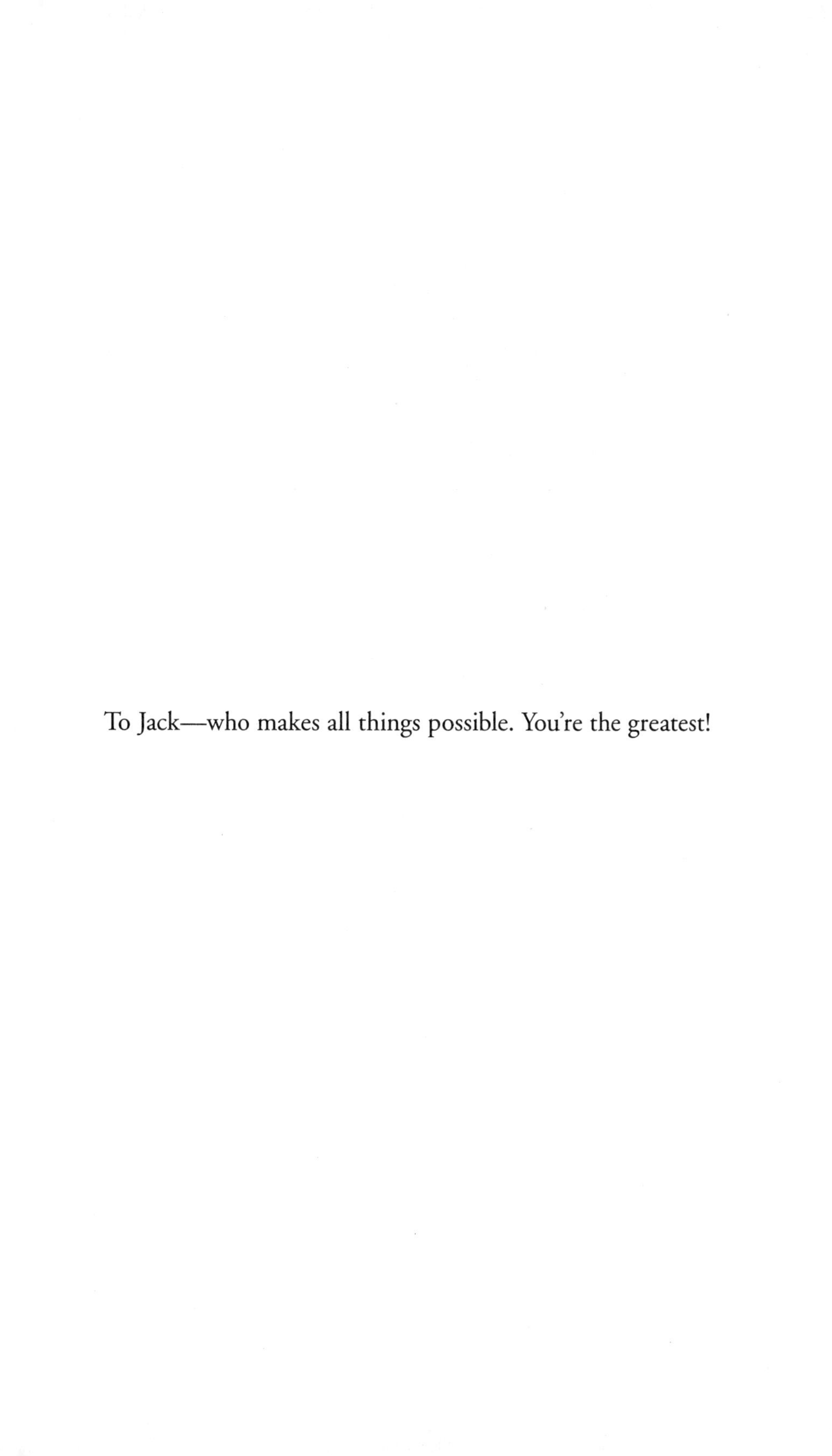

To Jack—who makes all things possible. You're the greatest!

Contents

Introduction

Aaachoo! Pass the tissues, folks, it's allergy season again. Here come the watery, itchy eyes; runny nose; coughing; sneezing and wheezing; postnasal drip; and endless fatigue that plague millions of Americans throughout the spring and fall—and sometimes during the summer, too. (Hey, that's 75 percent of the time!) And these are just the symptoms of seasonal allergies that affect the upper respiratory system. There are many other kinds of allergies, causing symptoms so diverse you might never guess they're the result of an overachieving immune system. For example, did you know that an allergy could be the culprit behind

- Anxiety, irritability, or panic attacks
- Joint and muscle pain or swelling of the extremities
- Attention deficit disorder, hyperactivity, lack of energy, or chronic fatigue syndrome
- Confusion, mental fatigue, or difficulty concentrating
- Congestion, difficulty breathing, or anaphylactic shock
- Depression
- Digestive upsets such as heartburn, gas, irritable bowel syndrome, colitis, nausea, vomiting, diarrhea, or constipation
- Heart palpitations, rapid heartbeat, or arrhythmia

- Insomnia, restlessness, early morning waking, oversleeping, or nightmares
- Rashes, hives, dermatitis, dry skin and hair, brittle nails, or eczema

It's tough enough dealing with the pollen, dust, and other natural substances that push our allergy buttons. Add to that the fact that the world around us is becoming more polluted, our water supply is being loaded with more and more additives, and our food supply is getting more refined and further from its natural state: it's not surprising that our bodies are rebelling. Let's face it, we were never designed to breathe, eat, and drink the cornucopia of chemicals we encounter every single day of our lives! And what do we do when we don't like our bodily reactions to these chemicals? We douse ourselves with even more chemicals in the form of drugs and medicines. Yet all we're really doing is temporarily suppressing our symptoms rather than treating the underlying causes. The real answer to curing allergies and asthma permanently doesn't lie in a doctor's little black bag or behind the pharmacist's counter. It can, however, be found in your own home, refrigerator, local gym, the offices of talented holistic healers, and in your own mind. You alone hold the keys to healing your allergies and asthma; nobody else can do it for you. As you'll see when reading this book, it might be easier than you think—although it requires some knowledge and plenty of persistence.

WHAT ARE ALLERGIES?

Allergies are the result of too much of a good thing or, to be more specific, your immune system working above and beyond the call of duty. The immune system—your "army within"—is absolutely vital to your health and well-being because it fights off the countless foreign bodies that invade your body every day. Specialized immune cells are able to identify the bacteria, viruses, and other unwelcome interlopers that take up residence inside you. The germs are first identified, then surrounded by an army of different kinds of immune cells that paralyze, disarm, or destroy them.

If your immune system is working well, disease shouldn't be able to get a permanent foothold. But when it can't distinguish between a true invader (like bacteria) and a harmless one (like pollen or dust), you're in trouble. That's because your immune system will wage war on things that aren't a threat, and you'll end up suffering all the symptoms of a real illness, like a cold or a rash or an upset stomach, without gaining anything. Your body is always the loser in these wars; valuable energy is wasted, normal tissue is damaged, bodily resources are drained, your immune system is depleted, and you suffer from symptoms that may drag on for months.

THE ALLERGIC REACTION

Normal, everyday substances in the environment that don't bother the average person can make the immune system of an allergic person declare war. These substances, called allergens, may seem as harmless as the dust on your dresser. But if you happen to be allergic to dust, it's not harmless at all. Let's say you've been cleaning out your attic, kicking up clouds of dust with each box of stuff that you move. As you breathe it in, your immune system improperly identifies this dust as an enemy. Warning bells go off, and your body starts to produce antibodies called immunoglobulin E, or IgE.

The immune system makes a special kind of IgE antibody for most allergens (including your particular brand of attic dust). These distinctive antibodies attach themselves to the surface of mast cells, the allergy-causing cells found in all the tissues in your body. These mast cells congregate in tissues that come in contact with the outside world, like the linings of the nose, throat, lungs, gastrointestinal tract, and reproductive organs. They contain loads of the chemical histamine, a high-powered inflammatory agent. Once your body produces a certain amount of IgE antibodies (in this case, antibodies to dust), the mast cells are primed to release their histamine. Then, the next time you breathe in a similar piece of dust, the mast cells will let loose with a flood of histamine that, in turn, triggers the inflammation response.

Nearby blood vessels become more porous, allowing their fluid and cells to seep out and flood nearby tissues. These tissues swell, becoming red, inflamed, and itchy. Mucus production may be stepped up in hopes of trapping the invaders and washing them away. And you're in the throes of a bona fide allergic reaction.

COMMON ALLERGENS

Just about anything can qualify as an allergen, but these are the most common:

- Chemical solvents
- Cosmetics
- Dander (a mixture of animal fur, skin scales, and saliva)
- Drugs
- Dust
- Dust mites (little animals that feed on dust and skin scales)
- Fabric
- Feathers or down
- Foods (see list on page xx)
- Fungi
- Fur
- Household cleaning products
- Medications
- Metals
- Molds
- Nuts
- Perfume

- Plastics
- Pollen
- Rubber
- Saliva (animal)
- Shellfish
- Smoke (tobacco)
- Venom

THE BUILD-UP EFFECT

Allergies aren't usually instantaneous; that is, it can take a while before you become allergic to something. Usually, the body won't release histamine and cause an allergic reaction until there's been a build-up of IgE antibodies to a certain substance. That's why you might have felt fine around your pet cat when you were a child, but as a teenager you suddenly couldn't go near her without getting a stuffy nose. This build-up effect may make each subsequent reaction worse, which is often the case with venom. (In certain people, each bee sting or snakebite causes more intense symptoms, culminating in anaphylactic shock, which can cause the closing of the airways, shortness of breath, convulsions, loss of consciousness, and even death.)

This build-up effect isn't always necessary, though—some substances can trigger an allergic reaction almost instantaneously. I remember getting a killer case of hives shortly after strolling across a vacant lot that had been sprayed with a highly toxic weed killer. And, conversely, the build-up effect can actually work in reverse—sometimes you actually grow out of certain allergies, especially if you're young. One thing is sure: it's practically impossible to predict the course that an allergy might take. It could get more intense, less intense, disappear completely, or only show up part of the time. (My mother never knows whether or not fresh pineapple is going to give her hives. She usually eats it and crosses her fingers!)

SYMPTOMS OF ALLERGIES

Your particular type of allergic reaction will depend on where the histamine is let loose in your body: whether it's in the skin, digestive tract, nasal passages, lungs, or elsewhere.

Skin Allergies

If histamine is released in your skin, that area may swell, itch, and develop red blotches, bumps, blisters, or other skin eruptions, all of which can be intensely irritating. Itching leads to scratching, which tears the skin and makes everything worse. Usually caused by exposure to chemicals, plants, cosmetics, toxins, or other environmental factors, allergies that affect the skin show up as one or more of the following:

- **Rashes** may appear as pinpoint, red spots; small, red, raised bumps; tiny blisters that ooze and crust; and so forth. They may cover the entire body or be confined to just one area. Rashes can be triggered by skin contact with allergens like chemicals, soaps, and perfumes.
- **Hives** are reddish-colored welts on the skin that itch like crazy and get worse when you scratch them. Hives can appear suddenly and disappear a few hours later, or they may last for days. Foods, insect bites, medicines, contact dermatitis, or stress can trigger them.
- **Contact dermatitis** may appear as skin redness, swelling, blisters, scaling, or crusting. Contact dermatitis occurs when the skin comes in contact with an allergen like poison ivy, cosmetics, deodorant, and so forth. A baby may develop contact dermatitis by wearing a diaper washed in a particular brand of detergent.
- **Eczema** often afflicts infants, causing redness, crusting, and oozing, usually of the face and scalp. In adults, affected patches are dry, red to grayish-brown, thickened and scaly, and typically appear on the elbows, back of the knees, wrists, ankles, face, and neck. Eczema

is usually a chronic condition, rather than a response to a single exposure to an allergen.

Allergies to Insect Venom

About 3 percent of us have immune systems that go completely out of control in response to the stings of bees, wasps, yellow jackets, or hornets, or to the bites of ants, mosquitoes, or fleas. Symptoms, which include headache, nausea, vomiting, coughing, stomach cramps, itchy skin, swelling of the face or throat, shortness of breath, and convulsions, can quickly progress to what's known as anaphylactic shock. If left untreated, it can be deadly.

Allergic reactions to insect venom tend to build with each subsequent sting or bite, becoming more dangerous and life-threatening. You can buy special emergency kits that contain epinephrine (the hormone adrenaline) in a syringe so that you can give yourself a shot immediately that will stop the reaction. See your doctor to get a prescription for this kit if you think you may be allergic to insect venom.

Allergic Rhinitis

When histamine is released in the nasal passages, you'll develop many of the symptoms of a head cold. Known to most of us as hay fever, *allergic rhinitis* literally means inflammation of the nasal passages due to allergens. (*Rhin* means nose, *itis* means inflammation.) But hay fever is actually a subcategory of allergic rhinitis, because it refers only to allergies caused by pollen. If you've got hay fever, you're already well aware that it strikes when the pollen is flying. Yet you don't have to be pollen-sensitive to suffer from allergic rhinitis. Dust, feathers, animal dander, mold spores (circulated courtesy of air-conditioning systems), and forced-air heaters that recycle dust can also do the trick.

Allergic rhinitis is responsible for the runny nose; itchy, watery eyes; sneezing; coughing; and postnasal drip that plague so many of us. It can also block the sinuses, giving rise to sinus headaches. Allergic rhinitis comes in two forms: seasonal, which typically occurs in the spring and in the fall, and perennial, which seems to go on forever (sort of like a head cold that never goes away).

Food Allergies

Histamine released in the digestive tract can cause stomach pain, nausea, vomiting, and diarrhea. The lips and tongue may start to tingle, then swell. But food allergies can also cause reactions that have nothing to do with the digestive tract. In fact, the first sign of an allergic reaction to a food is often a skin rash or hives. Food allergies aren't usually the culprit in respiratory trouble, such as asthma or hay fever, but in severe cases of food allergy, the body can go into anaphylactic shock. Luckily, that rarely happens.

The following foods are those most likely to cause allergies:

- Alcoholic beverages
- Caffeine
- Chocolate
- Citrus fruits
- Corn
- Dairy products
- Eggs
- Nightshade vegetables (tomatoes, eggplant, peppers, and so forth)
- Peanuts
- Shellfish
- Sugar
- Walnuts
- Wheat
- Yeast

Asthma

If histamine is released in your lungs, you can develop chest congestion and possibly asthma. Asthma, a growing problem, threatens our well-being in the most basic way: it cuts off our supply of oxygen. If you've got asthma, you're certainly not alone. As of 1998, there were 17 million self-reported cases of asthma in the United States, up from 14.6 million in 1994. And in the last ten years, the incidence of asthma in the United States has increased by a whopping 33 percent.

My husband Jack developed asthma when he was just seven years old. He spent a great deal of the second grade at home in bed and was rushed to the hospital gasping for breath on at least three occasions. Although he has since outgrown his childhood asthma, there are days when he suffers from a much milder form of the disease—that is, he just can't seem to get enough air with each breath and, as a result, feels very, very tired.

Because I don't have asthma myself, I had a hard time understanding what was happening to Jack. If he wasn't getting enough air, why couldn't he just take a bigger, deeper breath, the way you do when you're exercising? He tried to explain it to me. "The air can't get in," he'd say, but even he didn't know why.

I finally turned to some medical reference books and talked to a few doctors, and here's what I discovered. The respiratory system is like a large, upside-down tree. The trunk of the tree is your *trachea*, or windpipe; it branches into two smaller airways, called *bronchi*, each one leading to a lung. The bronchi then branch into even smaller airways, or *bronchioles*. Basically, both the bronchi and bronchioles are hollow tubes with muscular walls.

At the ends of the bronchioles, there are clusters of tiny air sacs, called *alveoli*, that are surrounded by capillaries. When you take a breath, the air is drawn all the way down into the alveoli, where the oxygen can slip through their very thin walls into the capillaries. Then it's whisked through the bloodstream to feed oxygen-hungry cells all over your body.

The reason you (or my poor Jack) just can't seem to get a decent breath during an asthma attack has to do with the faulty action of the bronchi and bronchioles. Three things happen:

1. The muscular walls of these tubes go into spasm, narrowing their passageways.
2. The linings of the tubes swell up.
3. The swelling of the tube linings makes them secrete extra mucus, which clogs the already-narrowed tubes.

Imagine your airways as a garden hose; the water that flows through represents your airflow. If you step on that hose, less water will be able to get through. Now suppose the inside lining of that hose suddenly swells up, and you also pour a jar of rubber cement down the hose. Your water flow will slow to a trickle, if any can get through at all.

Something similar happens when you have an asthma attack. You feel short of breath, there's a tightness in your chest, you wheeze, and you may cough a lot. You can find yourself sitting up, leaning forward, and using your neck and chest muscles to help you breathe. You get anxious, sweaty, and fatigued because the simple act of breathing is just so difficult. As it turns out, breathing out is even harder than breathing in, because when you relax your chest muscles (as you do when exhaling), your airways close up further. During severe asthma attacks, you may find yourself becoming drowsy and your lips might take on a bluish tinge due to a lack of oxygen. Asthma symptoms can run the gamut from life-threatening to mildly annoying and can last for minutes, hours, or even days.

Researchers believe that the spasms in the airways are often triggered by an allergic reaction to something that's been inhaled (e.g., pollen, animal dander, cigarette smoke, dust mites, mold, smog or other environmental pollutants, and so forth). But other things can trigger bronchial spasms, too: emotional stress, exercise, cold air, medications, infections, or anything else that irritates or stresses the airways. Normal, everyday things that wouldn't bother the average person can render an asthmatic breathless. Sometimes even a good, loud laugh will do it.

WHAT INCREASES YOUR CHANCES OF DEVELOPING ALLERGIES OR ASTHMA?

So why does one person get allergies or asthma, while another goes scot-free? Why does my husband Jack find himself short of breath when he walks past a freshly cut lawn, while I could take a nap on that same lawn with no problems at all? No one knows for sure, but heredity, diet, environment, and stress quite likely play major roles in determining who gets the honor.

Heredity

If either of your parents have allergies or asthma, you've got a good chance of developing them too. But it's not enough just to have, say, the "allergy gene." You also have to be exposed to factors that trigger the allergic response, and, in most cases, it takes repeated exposure.

Diet

A diet high in food additives, preservatives, and other chemicals may sensitize the body, making it more likely to develop allergic reactions. And if you're undernourished because, for example, you're getting too much animal fat but too little fiber, vitamins, and minerals, your body is going to be more likely to develop a whole range of diseases, asthma and allergies included.

Environment

Naturally, if you're sucking in a lot of smog, car exhaust, chemical fumes, air particulates, cigarette smoke, or other environmental pollutants, your lungs aren't going to be in great shape, and that can certainly predispose you to asthma. In fact, children whose mothers smoke more than ten cigarettes a day have twice the chance of getting asthma. It certainly makes sense to try to clean up your environment and stay away from pollutants, but if you're thinking of moving out to the country for its fresh air supply, you may want to think again. My friend Melinda moved to a beautiful little town in the mountains where the air is so clean and clear you can't help but drink it in. She was shocked when she found that her allergies flared up and just wouldn't simmer down. "It's the ragweed," she told me ruefully. "Who would have guessed that all this clean, pure mountain air would be worse for my allergies than city smog?" Her story reminds us that just cleaning up one element in your environment (in her case, the city smog), may not be enough, especially if you simply trade one allergen for another.

WHAT WESTERN MEDICINE DOES FOR ALLERGIES AND ASTHMA

The standard medical treatments for allergies and asthma are aimed more at getting rid of the symptoms than curing the disease. Antihistamines counteract the action of our body's natural "call to battle"—histamine—therefore calming the inflammation response. Decongestants and anti-allergy sprays shrink swollen nasal passages so that air can get through more easily. Synthetic steroid sprays also fight inflammation and help quell the allergic response. Bronchodilators relax the spasms in the bronchial tubes seen in asthma, and inhaled anti-inflammatory drugs ease inflamed membranes, opening airways even further.

These medications may be absolutely necessary to control your condition and, in some cases, may even save your life. But like all drugs, they also have side effects. Nasal sprays, for example, can become addictive and actually make nasal membranes even more inflamed over time. Antihistamines can cause drowsiness and interfere with your ability to drive, work, or operate machinery. Bronchodilators, drugs designed to open the airways, may cause rapid heartbeat, palpitations, or seizures. Cortisone can work wonders on allergic reactions, but long-term use can result in stomach bleeding, loss of calcium from the bones, cataracts, poor wound healing, weight gain, and mental problems.

While it may be absolutely essential for you to use medication to control your allergies or asthma, don't forget to look to Mother Nature for help in healing yourself. Natural remedies ranging from aromatherapy to Korean hand therapy, naturopathy to nutrition, and supplements to self-hypnosis can offer a kinder, gentler approach to easing your symptoms. At the same time, they work directly on the very things that either trigger your illness or make it worse (stress, environmental toxins, food additives, weak breathing apparatus, or poor general health). These remedies don't just mask your symptoms. Instead, they take a whole-body approach, treating your condition on more than just a physical level by addressing the emotional, mental, and spiritual realms, too.

BUT BEFORE YOU TRY ANYTHING . . .

Consult your physician before using any of the remedies described in this book, as some of them might actually make your condition worse, if your body is so inclined. Allergies and asthma can be life-threatening conditions that do require medication, so don't substitute natural remedies for medication without thoroughly discussing this with your medical doctor in advance.

HOW TO USE THIS BOOK

The most basic, effective, get-to-the-heart-of-the-matter ways to conquer the allergy/asthma problem are described in Chapters 1 through 10. These are also the safest and least likely to incite additional reactions. After you've worked your way through these, you may want to experiment with the natural therapies discussed in later chapters. Once again, be sure to consult with your physician first. When your immune system is constantly spoiling for a fight, you don't want to rile it up any further. Proceed with caution, but do try to keep an open mind.

1

Pinpoint the Triggers

The number-one way of relieving an allergy or asthma is to figure out what's triggering it, then avoid it. This sounds obvious, but it may not be as easy as you think, especially if your allergies are caused by "something in the air." The very first thing you need to do is analyze your symptoms so you can focus in on the kind of allergy you've got.

SYMPTOMS OF FOOD ALLERGIES

If you've experienced any of the following, especially after eating, you may have a food allergy:

- Rash or hives, involving part or all of the body
- Itchy, watery eyes or nose
- All-over itching
- Itching in the mouth or throat
- Nausea or vomiting
- Diarrhea
- Recurring earaches
- Anaphylaxis (swelling of the mouth, throat, or bronchial tubes that makes breathing difficult. Hives, swelling of the face,

wheezing, or fainting might also occur. Call 911 right away; this is a life-threatening reaction.)

SYMPTOMS OF SKIN ALLERGIES

A true skin allergy occurs when the skin comes in contact with an allergen and develops one or more of the following symptoms:

- Rash
- Swelling and itching of the skin
- Blisters
- Hives (red, raised patches on the skin)
- Rash that oozes and crusts

But the fact that you've got a rash doesn't necessarily mean you've got a skin allergy. You might get hives, for example, as a reaction to heat or eating too many strawberries (food allergy). But suppose, for example, you suddenly develop a rash on your arms after applying a particular lotion to them. Or if the area around you mouth gets red, bumpy, and itchy right after the dentist has worked on your teeth while wearing latex gloves. In these cases, you've probably got a skin allergy.

SYMPTOMS OF ALLERGY TO INSECT STINGS

The trigger for this one will be painfully obvious: when you've been stung by a bee or a wasp, you know it! All of us will experience at least a mild allergic reaction to insect venom; that's why we develop a raised welt, redness, itching, and irritation at the site. But those who are truly allergic to insect venom may develop an anaphylactic reaction, which causes airways to close and shock to set in. Symptoms leading up to this can include headache, nausea, vomiting, coughing, stomach cramps, itchy skin, swelling of the face or throat, shortness of breath, and convulsions. If you're suffering from anaphylaxis, use an emergency kit to give yourself an injection of epinephrine if possible, and get to the nearest emergency room immediately. If left untreated, anaphylactic shock can lead to death.

SYMPTOMS OF ALLERGIC RHINITIS

You might think you're suffering from a cold when you've really got an allergy. Symptom-wise, the difference between the two is that with an allergy your runny nose produces clear secretions instead of thick mucus.

The following symptoms may indicate allergic rhinitis (most commonly known as hay fever), especially if they occur seasonally or after exposure to substances like dust, animal dander, or pollen:

- Runny nose with clear secretions
- Sneezing
- Itchy nose and eyes
- Watery eyes
- Fatigue
- Asthma (allergy can bring on an attack)
- Symptoms that are worse in the morning

SYMPTOMS OF ASTHMA

Asthma, which literally means "to breathe hard," causes constriction of the airways and can produce symptoms that range from very mild to acute, including the following:

- Shortness of breath (difficulty in breathing, especially when exhaling)

- Exhalation that takes longer than inhalation (You feel the need to take another breath before you've finished exhaling the last one.)
- Wheezing (During exhalation, mucus in the airways causes a whistling sound.)
- Coughing (may be either a dry cough or a productive one; often it's the first indication that an asthma attack is coming on)
- Neck and chest muscles retract (an involuntary reaction to aid in the breathing process)

TESTS FOR ALLERGIES

Naturally, you'll want to see your doctor for a thorough diagnosis of your condition. Going to an allergist is probably your best bet, because a general practitioner may not recognize all kinds of allergies or be up on the latest treatments. The allergist will do various tests to pinpoint the allergens that are bugging you, including:

Blood Tests

A small sample of your blood is analyzed in the lab, checking for levels of certain antibodies, high white blood cell counts (an indication of an immune system reaction), or reactions between your blood and specific allergens.

Scratch Tests

Your skin is scratched, and a small amount of an allergen (in liquid form) is applied to the scratch. If a red, itchy bump appears, you're probably allergic to that allergen. The allergen can also be applied to the skin via a small patch for forty-eight to seventy-two hours.

Elimination Diets

The only way to find out if you've got a food allergy is to follow a strict diet that's made up of foods that almost never cause allergies, then add one food at a time and watch for reactions.

TESTS FOR ASTHMA

Breathing tests are used to measure lung function, confirm the diagnosis of asthma, and rule out other conditions. Two kinds of equipment are used: the peak flow meter and the spirometer.

Peak Flow Meter

This machine measures the speed of the air expelled during an exhalation, marking its fastest point. Because getting air out of the lungs is the major problem in asthma, the lower the speed of your exhalation, the more likely you are to be asthmatic. Another test that can be done with the peak flow meter is called the bronchial reversibility test. Your rate of exhalation is tested, then you're asked to use a bronchodilator (i.e., an inhaler) before being tested again. If your second score shows more than a 15 percent improvement, you may have asthma.

Spirometer

This machine measures the volume of air you can blow out of your lungs in one second. You take a big breath and blow it out into a tube as hard as you can. Normal lungs will expel about 70 percent of their air during the first second; those with asthma may blow out 50 percent or less.

WHAT TRIGGERS YOUR ASTHMA?

If your doctor should confirm that you do indeed have asthma, you'll need to do some digging to discover the causes. The most common trigger for asthma is allergies, especially in children. Allergens that are inhaled are particularly likely to set off an asthma attack—dust, animal dander, pollen, and mold—while food allergies rarely trigger an attack. Respiratory infections, strenuous activity, stress, emotional upset, cold weather, pollutants in the air, aspirin, ibuprofen, and sulfites (preservatives found in wine) can all bring on asthma attacks, so it's important that you analyze your environment, daily life, and attitudes in order to pinpoint the triggers.

Once you and your allergist finally zero in on what's bugging you, you can start to take positive steps to regain your health.

2

Reduce Allergens in Your Home

For those who suffer from asthma and allergies, the best offense is a good defense, especially at home where you have some control over your environment. If you can reduce or eliminate whatever seems to trigger your attacks, you'll be way ahead of the game. It's hard work, but can pay big health dividends. Consider the following suggestions for paring down the allergens in your home.

DECLARE WAR ON DUST

One of the worst allergens in existence is dust—or more correctly, the dust mite, a microscopic little animal that lives on dust and burrows into our pillows, mattresses, carpets, drapes, upholstered furniture, stuffed animals, and any other soft furnishings. These little mites leave droppings that float in the air; once we inhale them, the wheels of an allergic reaction can be set into motion. One mattress can harbor as many as two million of these little guys, and it's been estimated that 10 percent of the weight of a six-year-old pillow is due to dust mites, their waste, mildew, and mold. And whenever we walk across a carpet, clouds of dust mite droppings billow into the air—no wonder we get sick!

The best way to get rid of dust mites is to keep them from getting a foothold in your respiratory system in the first place. Special microporous covers should be placed over pillows and mattresses so dust mites can't get in or out; you can also buy pillows made with dust mite–proof barriers. Bedding should be washed every week in the hottest water; curtains and drapes should also be washed frequently. Don't use down-filled blankets or feather pillows; get hypoallergenic ones. Get rid of venetian blinds or miniblinds (they trap dust), and use shades instead. If you're highly allergic to dust, you may need to revamp your decorating scheme to do away with your carpets and drapes. And, sorry, but it's best to get rid of your stuffed animals. (If you just can't part with them, wrap them in plastic bags and freeze overnight to kill dust mites; then wash in 140°F water.)

Eliminate as much dust as possible—and you may find it helpful to wear a filter mask while you tackle these chores. When dusting furniture, use a cloth that's slightly damp so dust will be picked up instead of swept back into the air. Vacuum a lot (once a day, if necessary), and don't store things under your bed—they turn into dust-catchers that will also prevent you from vacuuming that area. Vacuums with microfilters are recommended (they suck up dust and don't let it loose), or you can buy microfiltration vacuum bags to fit the vacuum you have now. Either way, make sure you change your vacuum bag regularly—a full bag can throw more dust back into the environment than it picks up. You may also want to try a special allergen-removal product: Bissell has one called Multi-Allergen Removal Carpet Powder that you sprinkle on the carpet and vacuum up. They claim it will remove twice as many allergens as vacuuming alone.

A lot of dust is circulated via forced-air heating systems. If your heating system takes changeable filters, try using an electrostatic one. It's very effective and you won't have to buy replacement filters anymore, but you will need to clean it once a month to get rid of dust and pollen and keep it in working order. You might also try putting cheesecloth or an air-conditioner filter in each forced-air vent to keep out dirt, dust, and other irritants. These filters should also be changed once a month.

STAMP OUT SMOKE

You don't have to be a rocket scientist to know that smoke—whether from tobacco products, fireplaces, bonfires, or the food on your stove—is bound to make respiratory allergies and asthma worse. And studies have shown that a smoky environment can bring on these conditions in those who were previously unaffected, especially if they're children. Kids who regularly inhale secondhand smoke are twice as likely to become asthmatic, and many will develop chronic coughs, wheezing, and excessive phlegm. Pregnant women who smoke put their babies at a high risk of developing asthma and other respiratory problems.

Ban all forms of smoking in your home (cigarettes, cigars, marijuana, and anything else that produces smoke). Don't burn candles or incense, and avoid the use of wood-burning stoves or fireplaces. Gas stoves may also aggravate the symptoms of asthma, so you may want to look into getting an electric stove.

CAN THE CAT

All right, all right—maybe you can keep your cat, but if you're allergic to animal dander, you do so at your own risk! Cats are particularly allergenic, perhaps more so than any other animal, because of their grooming habits. They spend a good portion of the day licking their coats, cleaning off the dirt, grime, and loose hairs. Their saliva dries and releases a protein into the air that causes an allergic reaction in many people. You don't have to actually touch the cat or even be in the same room. In fact, this protein can remain in the house long after a cat has vacated the premises.

Animal dander refers to a mixture of skin scales and fur, and in cats, it also contains the salivary protein. But cats aren't the only culprits that cause allergic reactions—dogs, birds, or any other animal that has fur, hair, or feathers can do so, too. If you insist on keeping your pets, consider these guidelines:

- Keep pets off the furniture.
- Under no circumstances should you allow pets into your bedroom.
- Take furry animals to a professional groomer instead of trying to bathe them yourself.
- Get someone else to brush your furry animals frequently—outside! And store the brushes outside, too.
- Encourage pets to stay outside as much as possible.
- Wash your hands after handling pets.

MINIMIZE MOLD

Molds are a type of fungi that reproduce by forming spores that are released into the air. If a spore lands in a suitable environment, it takes root and grows into a new mold. Although millions of mold spores populate every cubic yard of air, only about twenty types cause allergies and asthma. Still, if one or more of those twenty happens to live in your house and you're sensitive to it, you can be headed for trouble. Mildew and aspergillus, for example, give off a harmful gas called benzene that can stir up allergic reactions.

Humidity is essential for molds to grow. Dripping taps; steamy bathrooms; old, musty papers and books; damp houses (especially in cellars); greenhouses; water beds; fish tanks; windows and windowsills; or compost heaps can foster the growth of mold, so these should be checked regularly. If possible, open the windows to increase ventilation—if this is not an option, try using a dehumidifier. Towel down the shower or bathtub after use. Wipe off condensation that gathers on windows, windowsills, and fish tanks, and be on the lookout for signs of black or green mold growth in damp areas. When you find it, scrub it away with a mixture of alcohol and lavender essential oil, or, in stubborn cases, use 50 percent chlorine bleach and 50 percent water. (Get someone else to do it for you if you can't handle chemicals.) Mold spores are often circulated courtesy of air-conditioning systems, but it can be difficult to clean the vents by yourself. Get a professional to check and clean your air-conditioning vents regularly.

HUNT DOWN HOUSEHOLD IRRITANTS

Although you might think your home is a haven from environmental pollution, chances are that once you walk in the front door, you exist in a virtual cloud of chemicals that make your allergies and asthma worse. Chemical solvents, household cleaning products, perfumes, cosmetics, hair spray, air fresheners, and fumes from gas stoves are just a few of them. And if you're a home improvement buff, you and your family have probably been exposed to the highly noxious chemicals found in spray paint and polyurethane varnish, plus those given off during soldering. Formaldehyde, which irritates the airways and eyes, is found in everything from paper to leather luggage.

So what should you do? First, keep your house well-ventilated. Our superinsulated homes with airtight windows and doors ensure that the same allergen-filled air is circulated over and over again. If the weather is agreeable, open the windows and get some fresh air going (unless it's pollen season and that's a problem for you). Use your air conditioner in warm weather, because it can help filter the air. Just make sure the vents stay clean.

Second, consider investing in an air-filtration system. The most effective are the high-efficiency particulate air (HEPA) filters. A HEPA filter traps 99.97 percent of all airborne particles that are 0.3 microns or larger, including dust, dust mite allergens, pollen, mold, animal dander, bacteria, and viruses. If you suffer from allergies or asthma because of airborne particles, a good air-filtration system may be your best friend.

Third, get rid of your harsh household chemicals. You can tackle your household cleaning chores by using a paste made from 2 parts baking soda and 1 part water for scrubbing, or a mixture of five tablespoons of white vinegar to one quart of water for cleaning windows and mirrors. (Save the chlorine bleach/water solution for really tough jobs.)

Finally, use cosmetics with caution. Most cosmetics come in hypoallergenic forms; always opt for these if you have a choice. Stay away from products that contain formaldehyde. Open the window when using hair spray. Roll-on deodorants are better for the environment (and you) than the spray kind. Stay away from perfume or products that contain perfume, because they contain irritants that inflame the airways and block sinuses. Unscented cosmetics are always preferable.

Although it will take time and energy to eradicate allergens from your home, it can be well worth the effort. Give it a shot!

3

Be Careful Outdoors

Ah, the great outdoors! Nothing is quite as invigorating as sucking up a lungful of fresh air; hiking through beautiful, flowering meadows; or taking a bike ride through the woods—unless, of course, you have allergies or asthma. Then the great outdoors can become one of your worst enemies, at least during certain times of the year.

POLLEN

Pollen is a major culprit when it comes to outdoor allergies. That fine, yellow dust that clings to the stamens of flowers and is transported from flower to flower on the legs of bees is also picked up by the wind and carried through the air. The pollen grain contains enzymes that help it penetrate the flowers; these enzymes also help it penetrate the lining of your nose and instigate an allergic reaction. And it's not just the pollen from flowers that can perform this little trick: grasses, trees, and plants also release their own forms of pollen that can trigger attacks. In fact, the major cause of allergies in the United States is ragweed pollen, a potent allergen found in large concentrations only there. During pollen season, a single ragweed plant makes and releases about one billion microscopic pollen grains, which can float through the air for hundreds of miles. The only places in the United States that aren't exposed to ragweed pollen are the southwestern desert areas and southern California.

In springtime, the major allergens come from trees, flowers, and grass. (My husband Jack often has trouble breathing when near a newly mowed lawn.) Breezy conditions make everything worse because more pollen becomes airborne, whereas on rainy days, pollen counts are usually low. In the summer, there may be tree and grass allergies, but allergic symptoms may ease because pollen from flowers is usually spread by insects rather than the wind during this time. But late summer and fall bring ragweed pollination, and that allergy, which lasts until the first frost, can be the worst of all.

If you're bothered by pollen allergies, consider these strategies for getting through the season:

- Keep your windows and doors closed as much as possible during pollen season.
- Use an air purifier to keep your indoor air as clean and pollen-free as possible.
- Stay inside as much as you can, especially during the early morning hours (peak pollen times) and on sunny, breezy days when pollen is likely to be flying.
- Use your home air conditioner to help filter the air.
- Drive with your car windows closed, and, again, use your air conditioner to filter the air.
- If you're very sensitive to pollen and must go outdoors during pollen season, wear a filter mask (like a surgical mask, available at hardware stores).
- Take your vacation at the beach, where offshore breezes tend to blow pollen inland, away from you.
- Avoid trips to the mountains, outdoor picnics, or camping during pollen season.
- Stay away from areas where long grass is growing.

- Wash your clothes and shampoo your hair after spending time outdoors.
- Exercise in the evening, when pollen counts are lowest.
- Wear sunglasses to protect your eyes from pollen grains.

To get daily pollen/spore counts for your city or general area, call the American Academy of Allergy, Asthma, and Immunology at 1-800-POLLEN or 1-877-9-ACHOO. Or you can visit their website, aaaai.org. Click on Patient/Public Resource Center, then National Allergy Bureau (NAB), then Pollen/Spore Counts. A map of the United States will pop up; click on your area and you can find a list of the type of allergens, their level, count, and even their history during the previous year.

ENVIRONMENTAL POLLUTION

You don't have to be living next door to a factory that billows noxious smoke for environmental pollution to aggravate your allergies. Smog, especially car exhaust, is a major source of trouble, producing chemicals like nitrogen dioxide, ground level ozone, benzene, and particulates, all of which irritate the lungs and aggravate breathing problems. Power plants spew sulfur dioxide, which constricts airways and contributes to the formation of acid air. Natural gas, pesticides, molds growing on rotting wood or leaves, animal by-products (especially urine), and wood dust can also wage war on your breathing apparatus and make you miserable. And breathing secondhand cigarette smoke not only makes asthma and respiratory allergies worse, but it can also cause cancer.

What do you do? First, treat heavily polluted days as you would heavy pollen days:

- Stay inside as much as possible.
- Keep doors and windows closed in both your home and car.

- Use air conditioners at home and in the car to filter the air.
- Exercise in the evenings when pollution levels are lower.
- Postpone activities that require heavy exertion.
- If you do exercise outside, wear a filter mask.

Then, consider these general guidelines for avoiding the effects of environmental pollution:

- Jogging or walking outdoors should be done away from heavy traffic areas.
- Don't live on a busy street, by a factory, or near a power plant.
- Wear a filter mask when cycling in traffic.
- Let somebody else do the house painting, fertilizing, or insecticide spraying.
- Don't go for walks in the woods or other moist places, especially during the fall, if you have a mold allergy.
- Avoid smoky areas such as bars, outdoor smoking areas, and campfires.

WEATHER

Although the weather itself isn't an allergen, there are times when it can bring on allergies or asthma. When a thunderstorm is brewing, pollen grains and spores are released into the air. The storm itself "inhales" a mixture of pollen, spores, and other pollutants; adds an electric charge; then deposits the whole mess on the ground along with the rain. People inhale these charged particles, which then stick to their lungs and cause asthma attacks. Hospital emergency rooms, in fact, often burst at the seams with asthmatic patients when thunderstorms strike. Although you certainly can't control the weather, do try to stay indoors as much as possible when you know a thunderstorm is brewing and continue to do so for a day or so after a storm has occurred.

HEAVY EXERCISE

Another trigger for asthma attacks is vigorous exercise, especially during cold, dry weather or at the height of pollen season. Exercise-induced asthma typically occurs in people who suffer from asthma at other times too, but there are some people who have asthma attacks only in response to exercise. It may only take five minutes of vigorous exercise to bring on an attack, and it usually happens after the exercise has stopped. If you suffer from exercise-induced asthma, don't go for a run or vigorously exercise outside on a cold, dry day or in the middle of pollen season. Stick to indoor activities instead.

INSECTS AND ANIMALS

What would the great outdoors be without plenty of animals, animal feces, insects, insect bites, and other things designed to make your allergies go crazy? Obviously, if you're allergic to animals or animal hair, fur, or feathers, you'll want to stay away from farms, corrals, petting zoos, chicken yards, and horseback-riding stables. Insects, however, can be a little trickier to avoid, so heed this advice, especially if you're allergic to insect venom:

- Always wear socks and shoes when you're outside.
- Wear a long-sleeved shirt tucked into long pants that are tucked into your socks, so insects can't fly up a pant leg.
- Gloves can also be a good idea, when gardening or when the weather is cool.
- Don't wear brightly colored fabrics, flowery prints, or sweet-smelling colognes or lotions. The bees may think you're a great big flower and zero in on you.
- Eating sweet foods attracts all kinds of insects—barbequed meats, fruit, candy, or ice cream draws them like magnets.

- Don't aggravate insects by swiping at them when they're buzzing around you—just walk away.

SUNLIGHT

Some people are actually allergic to the sun, a condition called photosensitivity. After just a few minutes of sun exposure, their skin may turn red, develop blisters or hives, and later begin to peel or form scaly patches. This is often caused by the use certain drugs or chemicals, such as antibiotics, preparations containing coal tar, perfumes, or scented soaps. Diseases like lupus (systemic lupus erythematosus) can also bring on photosensitivity. But in certain people, sun allergies are spontaneous and aren't linked to any other substance.

If you suffer from photosensitivity, you've got to be vigilant about covering up whenever you're anywhere near the sun. Consider these tips:

- Stay out of direct sunlight as much as possible.
- Remember that even if you're in the shade, reflected sunlight may cause a reaction. Staying indoors is safest, especially between ten A.M. and three P.M., when UV rays are most damaging.
- Use a high-protection sunscreen with an SPF of twenty or higher that shields against both types of ultraviolet radiation (UVA and UVB). The chemical compound that provides the best protection against UVA rays is avobenzone.
- Even more effective than chemical barriers are physical barriers to the sun, such as zinc oxide and titanium dioxide. These are the primary ingredients in the thick, white coating you've seen on the noses of lifeguards. Zinc oxide and titanium dioxide are available as opaque creams designed to cover especially sensitive areas such as the nose and lips, and are the primary ingredients in sunscreen lotions. (They may

leave a small amount of white residue, but they're the safest way to go if you've got a sun allergy.)

- Look for a sunscreen that does not contain para-aminobenzoic acid (PABA) or PABA derivatives, as these chemicals often irritate the skin.
- Apply sunscreen at least one-half hour before you go outdoors. Then reapply often (every two hours, or even more frequently if you're swimming or perspiring). Slather it on. Studies show that we usually put on far too little sunscreen.
- Wear sunproof clothing—thick fabric with a tight weave that doesn't let the light through.
- Wear long-sleeved shirts and skirts or pants that completely cover your legs.
- Avoid sandals—they expose too much skin. Shoes and socks are a better bet.
- A hat with a wide brim made of tightly woven material is essential.
- Get yourself a good pair of sunglasses that screen out both UVA and UVB rays.

Remember: "An ounce of prevention is worth a pound of cure." Other than staying indoors for the rest of your life, these tips are your best bet for dealing with Mother Nature without getting a mighty slap. Take heed—or be sorry!

4

Elimination Diet

A lot of people confuse the terms *food allergy* and *food intolerance.* My mother, for instance, always insisted that she was allergic to avocados. What happened to her when she ate avocados? She got an upset stomach. Sorry, Mom, but that's not an allergy; it's an intolerance.

In a true food allergy, eating a certain food (or sometimes just touching it or even being in the same room with it) triggers the immune system to wage war against this foreign invader. The heart may begin to pound, the breath comes harder and faster, the throat may swell causing choking, or a skin rash or hives might suddenly appear. Tremors, headache, fatigue, nausea, vomiting, diarrhea, and asthma attacks following ingestion of a particular food can all be signs of a food allergy. In some people, eating even a small amount of a certain food can produce anaphylactic shock, a major allergic response that can lead to death. Foods that are most likely to cause this reaction include peanuts, walnuts, pecans, milk, eggs, fish, shellfish, soybeans, and wheat.

The symptoms of food intolerance, on the other hand, tend to be much milder than those of food allergies. Stomach upsets (usually due to a deficiency in digestive enzymes such as lactase), a rise in blood pressure, sweating, headache, and spasms of the airways are common signs, but it usually takes a larger dose of the food in question to produce these symptoms. For example, my friend Leslie always gets a headache and rash after drinking two glasses of wine (it's the sulfites, a preservative in the wine), but if she keeps it to one glass, she's usually all right. That's a food intolerance.

Either way, if a food is producing a reaction (especially a big reaction), the best way to handle it is to avoid that food. That's fine if you happen to know which food or foods are offending your immune system. But if you don't, it's probably time to pay a visit to your friendly allergist. She will probably have you fill out a detailed questionnaire concerning your food habits, your history of allergies or asthma, the allergic reactions that run in your family, and so forth. There may also be a physical examination. The next step will probably involve the good old-fashioned elimination diet.

The idea behind the elimination diet is simple: begin by eating the blandest, least-allergenic diet possible, then slowly add different foods (except those that have already caused you to have an anaphylactic reaction) and wait for your body's response. If you get a rash, an asthma attack, or some other negative reaction, you're probably allergic to that food—or at least intolerant of it. Then, do your best to avoid eating it ever again. In some cases, it's possible that your body may grow out of a food allergy or intolerance, but taking shots or eating small amounts of the food and gradually increasing the dose usually won't cure you. The best idea is simply to stay away from the food.

START WITH THE LEAST OFFENSIVE FOODS

A typical elimination diet consists of foods that hardly anybody is allergic to—rice, fruits (non-citrus), vegetables, and unprocessed meat or poultry. Make sure you eliminate the "usual suspects," foods that commonly cause allergies:

- Alcoholic beverages
- Caffeine

- Chocolate
- Citrus fruits
- Corn and corn products
- Dairy products
- Eggs
- Food additives and preservatives
- Fruits
- Meat, meat products
- Nightshade plants (eggplant, peppers, potatoes, tomatoes)
- Peanuts
- Shellfish
- Soy products
- Sugar
- Tree nuts (walnuts, pecans, and so forth)
- Wheat and wheat products
- Yeast

Some people have found that the food that causes an allergic reaction is either the one they eat the most or the one they crave the most, like chocolate or wheat products. It may help to keep a detailed food diary, recording the food you eat, any symptoms that occur, how long it takes before the symptoms show up, and how much food it takes to produce a reaction.

Make up your own elimination diet, eating the least allergenic foods and avoiding any that you think might be causing your symptoms. Follow this diet for two weeks. If you're still having symptoms after that, restrict it further, following the guidelines above, and consult your allergist.

SLOWLY ADD THE "USUAL SUSPECTS"

Once you're free of food-allergy symptoms, it's time to begin the test. Get somebody to help you with this, because you shouldn't know in advance which food is being reintroduced into your diet, or even if you're getting a new food at all. A small amount of the food (one-half to one teaspoon) should be mixed into a food that's already part of the elimination diet. Some days nothing should be added, to see if a reaction might be psychologically induced. As long as no reaction is detected, the amount of the food in question should be increased over a two-week period until it resembles a normal-sized portion. (Obviously, after a while you'll know you're getting the food since it can no longer be disguised within another food.)

When you've determined the status of one food, repeat the process with the next food. As you can imagine, this is a rather long, painstaking procedure, especially if you're testing a lot of foods. But it's essential that you stick faithfully to the plain foods in the elimination diet. Adding in several foods at once or eating mixed foods (e.g., bread, cake, casserole, sandwiches, and so forth) can make it impossible for you to know what's causing a reaction.

ONCE YOU KNOW WHAT YOU'RE ALLERGIC TO . . .

Be on the lookout for the foods that trigger your allergies. This is harder than it might seem, because we often don't know what we're eating. Become an avid label reader, don't be afraid to question waiters or others in the food service business, and take a good look at what you're about to eat. This isn't absolutely vital if your problem is simply a food intolerance, or even a mild allergy. But if you happen to have an anaphylactic reaction to certain foods, it can mean the difference between life and death. My sister-in-law Fienie goes into anaphylactic shock if she eats walnuts, which can show up in just about everything—casseroles, brownies, cookies, even salad. She has to look carefully at what she eats and ask questions, or she'll be in big trouble. It's a pain, but for her it's the only solution.

5

Eat Defensively

Our food supply is certainly plentiful, but it's far from safe if you have a tendency toward allergies and asthma. Some 3,500 additives are hidden within the foods we eat, and although not too many will trigger out-and-out allergic reactions, some can cause symptoms that range from the annoying to the downright dangerous. If you have allergies or asthma that may be food-related, you'll need to be cautious about what goes into your mouth. That can be a tough job, admittedly, but your dedication might make a decided difference in your health.

AVOID FOOD ALLERGENS

Obviously, you should stay away from foods that you know will trigger allergic or asthmatic reactions in your body. But you should also avoid foods that are common allergens unless you know for a fact that they don't bother you. Chances are if you're allergic to one thing, you're probably allergic to at least a couple more. These are some of the foods that cause allergies or asthma in many people:

- Alcoholic beverages
- Caffeine
- Chocolate
- Citrus fruits
- Corn and corn products
- Dairy products
- Eggs
- Food additives and preservatives
- Fruits
- Meat, meat products
- Nightshade plants (eggplant, peppers, potatoes, tomatoes)
- Peanuts
- Shellfish
- Soy products
- Sugar
- Tree nuts (walnuts, pecans, and so forth)
- Wheat and wheat products
- Yeast

See Chapter 4 for tips on how to use an elimination diet. This will help you to determine whether or not these foods pose a problem for you.

WATCH OUT FOR INFLAMMATORY FOODS

Some foods promote the inflammation response, so try to keep away from these:

- Vegetable oils that are high in omega-6 fatty acids (corn, safflower, and sunflower seed oils)
- Animal fat
- Beef, especially heavily marbled

STEER CLEAR OF PRESERVATIVES AND ADDITIVES

Fast food; restaurant fare; canned, frozen, or processed foods: the things that many of us put into our bodies every day are littered with chemical additives and preservatives. Always try to eat food in its natural state, if possible (fresh, raw vegetables and fruits; cooked whole grains; lightly broiled meat, fish, or poultry; and so forth). If you do eat processed foods (and who doesn't, at least some of the time?), try to avoid the following:

Aspartame

This artificial sweetener, found in soft drinks, chewing gum, and candy, can cause hives, headaches, and inflammation responses in certain people. If you want to eat something sweet, reach for dried fruit, honey, or even sugar—at least it's not some conglomeration of chemicals born in a laboratory.

BHA/BHT

These synthetic antioxidants are added to salad dressings, cake mixes, cereals, crackers, and grain products to keep fats from going rancid. But they may cause rashes, headaches, and, in children, hyperactivity. Make your own salad dressing and cake from fresh ingredients; buy baked goods or crackers without preservatives and store them in the freezer to keep them fresh.

Chlorine

This is routinely added to tap water, along with other chemicals, to keep our water supply safe. Many cities also add fluoride to help prevent tooth decay. If you're allergic to any of these chemicals, however, better stick to bottled spring water instead.

Food Coloring and Dyes

These additives may play a major part in attention deficit disorder and hyperactivity, hives, bronchial congestion, and digestive upsets. Eat fresh and unprocessed foods, right off the tree if possible, and you won't need food coloring because the food is already at its most colorful and appealing.

Ethylene Gas

Sprayed on bananas to speed up their ripening, ethylene gas may trigger an asthmatic reaction in certain people. Buy organic bananas and let them ripen naturally.

Monosodium Glutamate (MSG)

Found in Chinese food, meat tenderizer, and a host of processed foods, MSG may bring on asthma, diarrhea, tightness of the chest, and migraine headaches. Try making your own Chinese food by stir-frying fresh vegetables along with small amounts of meat or poultry. It's better than takeout, and you won't wind up with a migraine!

Nitrates/Nitrites

These preservatives, found primarily in cured or processed meats such as hot dogs, bacon, ham, and bologna, may cause hives, headaches, digestive upsets, and blood pressure problems. Once again, stick to fresh meats that you cook yourself.

Pesticides

Sprayed routinely on the produce we buy in the grocery store, insecticides, herbicides, and fungicides may trigger symptoms of asthma. Look for organic produce that has been grown without the aid of pesticides. If you can't find it, wash your vegetables and fruits in a large basin of cold water to which you've added one tablespoon chlorine bleach (this will act as a soap). Then rinse it off with plenty of cold water.

Sulfites

A preservative found in certain wines and used to keep vegetables from turning brown, sulfites can cause allergic reactions like wheezing, difficulty breathing, vomiting, diarrhea, hives, and dizziness. The law requires that the presence of sulfites be clearly stated on the food label, so read those labels as if your life depended on it. And be careful in restaurants, where vegetables may be treated with chemicals to keep them fresh. Salad bars are particularly notorious for bathing their vegetables in sulfites so they won't turn brown. You're better off eating at home, where you know what's in your food.

EAT "ANTI-INFLAMMATORY FOODS"

"Okay," you must be saying. "Don't eat this, that, or the other thing. Is there anything I *can* eat?" Luckily, the answer is yes. Certain foods have ingredients that help fight the inflammation response and alleviate congestion; itchy, watery eyes, runny nose; and inflamed bronchial tubes. They include:

- Fish high in omega-3 fatty acids (albacore tuna, salmon, mackerel, sardines, herring, sablefish, rainbow trout, to name a few)
- Fruits and vegetables, especially those high in vitamin C
- Onions
- Garlic

Be sure to include these foods in your meals as often as you can for the best protection against future attacks.

"I'LL TAKE ONE LATTE WITH A DASH OF CHILI PEPPER"

Here's good news for all of you who like your food as hot and spicy as you can get it. Hot peppers and spicy foods can help open up air passages. So, if you like jalapeño peppers, horseradish, or supercharged hot sauce that makes the steam come out of your ears, go for it!

Coffee lovers with asthma will be happy to hear that a cup of good, strong coffee may be an antidote to asthma attacks because caffeine dilates the bronchial tubes. One study of twenty thousand Americans revealed that those who drank coffee on a regular basis had 33 percent fewer asthma symptoms than those who didn't drink coffee at all. They were also significantly less likely to suffer from bronchitis, wheezing, and allergies. One cup a day is good, but three cups appear to be even better.

EAT WISELY AND WELL

Finally, try to eat a balanced diet to keep your body strong and less susceptible to allergies or asthma. This can be tricky if you're allergic to entire groups of foods, like dairy foods. But do your best to approximate the following:

- **Six to eleven servings of grain products per day (whole grain bread, cereal, rice, pasta)**—If you have an allergy to wheat or other grains, try rice products, which are the least allergenic.
- **At least five servings of fruits and vegetables**—Fresh is best; avoid canned or frozen as the linings of metal cans or plastic bags may cause allergic reactions.
- **Two to three servings of meat, fish, poultry, eggs, dry beans, or nuts**—This is the group most likely to cause allergies, so only eat foods from this group that your body can tolerate.
- **Two to three servings of milk, cheese, or yogurt**—Some people may have an asthmatic reaction to milk. If you've got asthma, go

easy on the milk and watch for symptoms. If, for whatever reason, you can't tolerate dairy foods, take a calcium supplement instead (800 to 1,000 milligrams per day for most people; 1,500 milligrams for postmenopausal women).

- **Fats, oils, and sweets**—Add in limited amounts only for flavoring.

Vary your selections from day to day within each food group. Food can be like clothes—you tend to eat (or wear) the same things over and over again. But you may have developed allergies to some of these foods, and you'll never know it until you stop eating them.

6

Attack Allergies with Supplements

Doctors have not yet invented the "allergy-be-gone" pill that my allergic-to-everything husband Jack yearns for, but there are lots of "little pills" that may be able to nibble away at your tendency to suffer from allergies and asthma and their bothersome symptoms. These little pills are vitamins, minerals, and other supplements, most of which are readily available from your local grocery or health food store.

VITAMINS

Here's a list of what certain vitamins can do to ease your allergies and asthma.

Beta-Carotene

Beta-carotene is the plant form of vitamin A, but once it's inside our bodies it is converted to the latter form. In either incarnation, it performs important functions. Beta-carotene is linked to an increase in the body's ability to fight infection, while vitamin A plays a crucial role in the maintenance of healthy mucous membranes, skin, eyes, lungs, and connective tissue, among other things. It's a fact that those who have low blood levels of vitamin A typically have more upper respiratory infections. A daily dose of 25,000 I.U. of beta-carotene is often recommended to help your body fight off invaders and maintain healthy tissue.

Vitamin B_3 (Niacin)

Way back in 1944, people suffering from bronchial asthma or hay fever improved rapidly after being given shots of niacinamide, a form of niacin. That's because niacinamide inhibits the release of histamine, the substance that sets off the whole process of inflammation or congestion. Niacin itself can help reduce wheezing. A 1990 study, reported in the *Journal of Clinical Nutrition*, found that the amount of niacin a person consumes and the levels of niacin in the blood are inversely correlated with the amount of wheezing asthmatics do. In other words, the higher the niacin levels, the less wheezing. A 25 to 50 milligram dose per day is often recommended.

Vitamin B_5 (Pantothenic Acid)

A contributing factor to the production of cortisone (a natural anti-inflammatory) and other adrenal hormones, pantothenic acid is used to support adrenal gland function. A daily intake of 4 to 7 milligrams is often recommended.

Vitamin B_6

This vitamin may help reduce the symptoms of asthma in children. A report in the *Annals of Allergy* described a study involving seventy-six children with moderate to severe asthma. The children were divided into two groups: one was given 200 milligrams of B_6 daily, the other a placebo. Five months later, the youngsters who had been given the vitamin had far fewer asthma symptoms and were taking fewer medicines. B_6 can also help guard against "Chinese restaurant syndrome." Otherwise known as hypersensitivity to MSG, this syndrome can cause a runny nose, headache, or other problems after one consumes the MSG often found in Chinese food. In one study, people who were taking B_6 regularly had fewer reactions after eating foods containing MSG. Experts often recommend 25 to 200 milligrams of this vitamin, daily.

Vitamin B_{12}

Found only in foods that come from animals (meats, poultry, eggs, fish, and so forth), vitamin B_{12} might reduce the symptoms of contact dermatitis and sulfite allergies. A 1951 study in the *Journal of Allergy* reported that six patients with contact dermatitis improved when given weekly injections of B_{12}. And in the 1980s, it was discovered that B_{12} taken sublingually (under the tongue) helps guard against reactions to the sulfites used to preserve fresh vegetables and wines.

Vitamin B_{12} can also help reduce wheezing, especially in children. Long before many of our modern medicines were introduced, doctors knew that large doses of this vitamin injected right into the muscle helped reduce the symptoms of asthma, particularly in the young. The idea of using B_{12} to treat asthma was reintroduced in 1989. In a study of the vitamin involving some fifty children under the age of ten, 60 percent completely stopped wheezing, and another 20 to 30 percent enjoyed significant relief. An often-recommended dosage is between 9 and 25 micrograms, daily.

Vitamin C

Doses of 2,000 milligrams, daily, spur the release of antihistamines, which help ease allergic reactions as well as congestion of the nasal passages, sinuses, and bronchial tubes. But doses of this size may also cause diarrhea, stomach cramps, and drying of the nasal passages. (To avoid these unpleasant side effects, 1,000 milligrams, twice a day, is often recommended instead.)

Vitamin C has also been linked to fewer asthma symptoms. Looking at data from the massive National Health and Nutrition Examination Surveys (NHANES), researchers found that the more vitamin C people consumed in their food and the higher the vitamin C levels in their blood, the less likely they were to suffer from wheezing or other lung problems. Scientists in Scotland looked at people who had breathing difficulty that was related to the seasons (e.g., asthma in the spring and fall). Those who had the lowest intakes of vitamin C had five times the breathing difficulty of those who had the highest intakes.

Several other studies have also shown that taking vitamin C can reduce the number of asthma attacks one suffers and make it less likely to suffer one after exercising. Doses of between 500 and 2,000 milligrams, daily, are often recommended.

Vitamin E

This well-known free radical quencher infiltrates the fatty membrane of cells and protects them from damage, particularly the oxidation of their fats. Vitamin E is also a great neutralizer of ozone, a major part of smog that wreaks havoc on the respiratory system and makes asthma and allergies worse. Recommended doses typically range from 400 I.U. to 1,000 I.U. of vitamin E, daily.

MINERALS

Minerals play important roles in body structure, the makeup of certain compounds, and the regulation of body processes. But they can also help calm allergic reactions and sometimes even prevent those reactions from occurring in the first place. The minerals that may be most helpful include the following.

Calcium

This mineral, a major part of our bones and teeth, can also help reduce allergic reactions in the skin and respiratory tract. Long used to treat these problems, calcium was finally put to the test in a study done in 1993. Researchers found that a daily dose of 1 gram (1,000 milligrams) of supplemental calcium significantly reduced the swelling of the nasal mucosa caused by allergens. Another study showed that calcium plus vitamin D_2 helped ease airway constriction in asthma.

Magnesium

Magnesium sulfate is a natural bronchodilator, relaxing the smooth muscle in the bronchial tubes. (Many hospitals use it intravenously to treat asthma attacks.) Although taking magnesium tablets won't have the immediate effects seen with intravenous magnesium, it may help reduce wheezing and can be helpful over time. The recommended dose is usually 500 milligrams, per day. Don't exceed 1,000 milligrams, daily.

Selenium

Asthma has been linked to low blood levels of this important antioxidant, and one study showed that asthmatics improved significantly when taking selenium supplements. Selenium helps maintain the health of cell membranes and fights free radical damage to cells and tissues. Doses of 50 to 200 micrograms, daily, are generally recommended; more than 200 micrograms, daily, could be toxic.

OTHER SUPPLEMENTS

Certain substances besides vitamins and minerals may also be helpful in controlling asthma or allergies, including the following.

Bromelain

This enzyme comes from the pineapple and blocks inflammation by producing a substance that breaks down fibrinogen, which plays a part in swelling. Bromelain is also good for the digestion—exerting just the opposite effect of certain over-the-counter anti-inflammatory drugs. One to three 500-milligram tablets, per day, are generally recommended.

Methylsulfonylmethane (MSM)

A form of organic sulfur that is easily absorbed by the body, MSM is used to make antibodies, antioxidants, enzymes, connective tissue, and amino acids. Some studies have shown that MSM effectively quells even the severe symptoms of allergies and asthma. Especially when combined with vitamin C and bioflavonoids, MSM can get rid of watery eyes, runny nose, sneezing, and congestion in just a couple of weeks. Organic sulfur is also nonallergenic, unlike sulfa drugs, which can cause severe reactions in some people. The recommended dosage is generally 1,000 milligrams, twice a day, with food.

Omega-3 Fatty Acids

Researchers looking at what people eat found a link between the consumption of fish oil (which contains the omega-3 fatty acids) and wheezing and bronchitis. It seems that the more fish oil consumed, the fewer asthmatic symptoms experienced. This is probably because omega-3 fatty acids have a natural anti-inflammatory effect that helps quell the major symptoms of both asthma and allergies. Researchers have also found that besides calming the initial inflammatory phase of asthma, fish oils also slow or halt the late-phase reaction—one that occurs as much as twenty-four hours later and may be the cause of chronic asthma and damage to the tissues.

Like certain fish, flaxseed oil is also a good source of omega-3 fatty acids. The generally recommended dose of fish oil is six 1,000-milligram capsules, daily, for those who eat fish; or up to twelve for those who don't eat fish. For flaxseed oil, good results can be obtained from 3 tablespoons per day or the equivalent in capsules. (Don't take both oils and don't take more than the recommended dosage of either, because the omega-3s are blood thinners and can interfere with normal blood clotting. And be sure to speak to your physician before taking omega-3 fatty acids if you're on blood-thinners or other medication.)

Quercetin

Found in Italian squash, grapes, and yellow and red onions, this bioflavonoid is an excellent anti-inflammatory. It slows down the release of histamines, which cause the sneezing, sniffling, and congestion found in allergies. It also interferes with the release of leukotrienes, substances that bring on asthmatic reactions. Unless you already eat the equivalent of one red or yellow onion daily, your health advisor may suggest 400 milligrams of quercetin, daily, as a preventive measure.

Rutin

Another of the bioflavonoids, rutin is necessary for vitamin C absorption. Like quercetin, it works to slow the release of histamine. It's also an anti-inflammatory that fights both bacteria and viruses. Because it's so effective, rutin is included in many anti-allergy formulas that you can buy off the shelf. The recommended dosage is often 500 milligrams, daily, between meals.

SUMMING IT UP

Supplements are a good idea, since few of us eat really well. You can get most of the above nutrients by taking a multivitamin/multimineral, plus the major antioxidants: vitamins A (beta-carotene), C, E, and selenium. If you've got asthma, you may want to ask your doctor about adding a moderate amount of fish oil or flaxseed oil. Whatever you do, remember that when you start taking supplements, it's wise to start with the lowest dose and watch carefully for reactions.

7

Strengthen Your Lungs with Breathing Exercises

We've all been breathing since the obstetrician held us up by our feet and gave us that first spank, so you'd think we'd know what we're doing by now! But an amazing number of us—as many as 25 percent—don't know how to breathe properly. We breathe shallowly, using only the top half of our lungs rather than filling our lungs to their full capacity. As a result, we can hyperventilate, and that may lead to fatigue, stress, tension, poor physical performance, headaches, and sometimes even asthma.

You can take air into your body and expel it in two basic ways: using your chest or using your diaphragm, a dome-shaped muscle that sits between your chest and abdominal cavities. During proper breathing, as you pull air into your lungs your diaphragm will flatten out to give your lungs more room to expand. The chest expands somewhat, but the major action occurs in the diaphragm. Breathing from the diaphragm allows your lungs to fill to capacity and is the best way to fully oxygenate your body. But many of us are die-hard chest-breathers, that is, we breathe shallowly using just the top half of our lungs. Most of the action centers in the upper chest and the muscles of the rib cage. Chest-breathing is the kind of breathing you do when you're stressed out or very excited about something. Your breath starts coming faster and harder. While your heart may be beating more quickly during chest-breathing, you are not getting as much oxygen per breath as you would be if you were breathing from your diaphragm.

If you tend to be a chest-breather, you may be exacerbating your asthma. You also may be adding to the tension and stress in your life. The exercises that follow will help you learn to breathe more efficiently and can help east fatigue, stress, and the severity of your asthma attacks.

BREATHING FROM THE DIAPHRAGM

This exercise is designed to teach you the difference between breathing from the chest and breathing from the diaphragm. You can use this technique just about anywhere: while sitting at your desk, driving a car, watching television, or before going to bed. It's wonderfully relaxing and energizing, and it's a great conditioner for your lungs.

1. To begin, lie on your back with legs extended or with knees bent and feet flat on the floor, whichever feels more comfortable. Or, you may sit erect in a chair. Your arms should be at your side. Take a moment to relax completely.
2. Place your hands lightly over your diaphragm, which is located just below your rib cage, directly underneath your sternum.
3. Inhale slowly and deeply to a count of 5, inflating your diaphragm area and using it to push your hands as high as they will go. Keep your chest muscles and shoulders as relaxed as possible. All the work should come from the diaphragm.

4. Exhale by contracting your diaphragm area and slowly pushing the air out. Make sure you breathe out every last little bit of air. Exhalation is even more important than inhalation because it clears the way for the entrance of new, oxygen-rich air.
5. When you think you've exhaled every last bit of air, try to make a humming sound. You may be surprised to find that you still have enough air to manage to hum for another count or two!
6. Repeat this exercise several times. Do it slowly, completely filling and emptying your lungs each time. When you've mastered the technique in a lying-down position, try it sitting up with your legs tucked underneath you.

THE FLICKERING CANDLE

Controlling your breath and exhaling completely are the essential elements in this exercise.

1. Light a candle and sit in front of it, back straight, shoulders relaxed, and hands lying limp in your lap. The flame of the candle should be about the same height as your mouth, so either cut the candle down or place some books underneath it to adjust it to this position.
2. Take some slow, deep breaths to relax.
3. Inhale fully, purse your lips, and slowly expel the air, causing the candle flame to flicker but not go out completely.
4. When you have completed your exhalation, relax your lips, and inhale slowly through your nose.
5. Take a few more slow, deep breaths before repeating.

The point of this exercise is to learn to control your breath: don't let it all out in a big rush, but keep releasing just enough to make the flame waver.

THE HURRICANE

While The Flickering Candle is good for breath control, The Hurricane helps increase the strength and velocity of your exhalation.

1. Light a candle and sit in front of it, as you did in The Flickering Candle exercise.
2. Inhale deeply, using your diaphragm.
3. Purse your lips and blow the air out as hard and fast as you can, making every attempt to blow out the candle.
4. Slowly inhale and take a few more slow, deep breaths before repeating.

ALTERNATE NOSTRIL BREATHING

This yoga breathing exercise (called a *pranayama*) is designed to increase the power of your exhalation.

1. Sit on the floor with your back erect in a cross-legged position.
2. Touch the bridge of your nose with the thumb and index finger of your right hand.
3. With your middle finger, press on the outside of your nose, closing your left nostril.
4. Through your open right nostril, breathe in and out rapidly and forcefully, 8 to 10 times.
5. Using your left hand and left nostril, repeat.

THE CONTROL PAUSE

The brainchild of a Russian scientist named Konstantin Buteyko, The Control Pause is both a method of measuring the effectiveness of your breathing and a way of controlling hyperventilation.

1. Sit in a chair, relaxed but back erect.
2. Exhale completely, then breathe in gently.
3. Exhale once again and hold your nose with your thumb and index finger so no air can enter.
4. Using a stopwatch, note the length of the "control pause" (the amount of time that you can last before taking another breath). One minute = terrific; 40 to 60 seconds = good, healthy lungs; 30 seconds = mild asthma; 10 seconds = severe asthma.
5. To use this method as an exercise, perform the control pause 6 times each day: 4 times aiming to hold your breath as long as you can, and 2 times trying to hold it for half that length of time. Use this pattern: 2 maximum, 1 half-max, 2 maximum and 1 half-max, with 3-minute breaks in between each control pause.

Proponents of this method claim that you can use it to stop an asthma attack in its tracks, and that after just a couple of days of practicing you may be able to cut your medication back 40 to 100 percent.

Breathing exercises are an absolute must-do for those with asthma and not a bad idea for everyone else. Increase your breathing capacity and you will automatically increase your energy and boost your health.

8

Get Fit!

Exercise and allergies have never been mutually exclusive. If you have allergies and want to exercise, you simply need to bear in mind what you're allergic to and avoid it (e.g., don't jog through a meadow at the height of pollen season, don't ride your bike in the murky wake of bus exhaust, and take along a bee sting kit). But exercising with asthma can be another story. Although exercise is certainly good for overall health, vigorous exercise can bring on an asthma attack (a condition called *exercise-induced asthma*), or make an existing attack worse. Those with exercise-induced asthma may cough, wheeze, or feel unable to catch their breath shortly after they begin exercising. Or these symptoms may not show themselves until after the exercise session is over. Luckily, most exercise-induced asthma attacks aren't the acute kind that allergens can sometimes trigger.

EXERCISE: A BETTER FRIEND THAN ENEMY

In the past, we thought that asthmatics were better off if they were sedentary and didn't push themselves physically. The stereotypical asthmatic child was one who sat quietly on the sidelines, a thin, pale shadow of his more robust classmates, who ran and shouted boisterously as they played their games. But today we know that sitting on the sidelines and conserving one's energy is not the ideal solution. That's because getting and staying physically fit are two of the best ways to combat just about any disease or ailment, including asthma. Exercise strengthens the respiratory system and increases lung capacity, so breathing becomes easier. It also strengthens the cardiovascular system, improving the efficiency of both the heart and the circulation, while lowering blood pressure and decreasing the blood fats that can cause heart disease. Exercise also builds muscles, burns excess fat, relieves stress, improves the quality of sleep, and just plain makes you feel better.

With all of these benefits, experts say it's important to include exercise in your life, even if you do have asthma. The trick is to know your limitations and not try to push yourself too far, too fast. Things that you should take into consideration when setting up an exercise program include:

- First and foremost, see your physician before beginning or expanding any exercise program, and follow his or her guidelines.
- Start slowly with mild exercise, especially if you haven't done anything in awhile. Walk instead of run, cycle on flat ground instead of hills, or swim at a relaxed pace instead of a fast one.
- Be careful about exercising outdoors during cold, dry weather because it can trigger asthma attacks.
- Avoid allergens like pollen, mold, and dust. (See Chapter 3 for other cautions about outdoor exercising.)
- If you feel an asthma attack coming on, stop exercising and relax.
- If you have medication for your asthma, take it before exercising and bring it along with you for emergency assistance.

THE FIVE ELEMENTS OF A GOOD EXERCISE PLAN

There are five elements to every good exercise plan.

1. **Warm-up**—Always warm up your muscles at the beginning of your exercise session to get your circulation going and to raise the temperature in your muscles. This will get your body ready for heavier exercises and help prevent injuries. Brisk walking or light calisthenics are good warm-up exercises.
2. **Cardiovascular endurance exercises**—These are commonly known as *aerobic* exercises, a Greek word that means "with air." They're called that because these exercises require a good air supply, and they do get you to breathe more rapidly and deeply, while speeding up your heart rate. Cardio exercises include fast-paced walking, jogging, running, cycling, dancing—anything that revs up your heart and makes you huff and puff a little bit. These are great for increasing your lung capacity, toning up your cardiovascular system, and burning excess fat.
3. **Strengthening exercises**—These exercises build and tone your muscles, bones, tendons, and ligaments by forcing your body to work against some form of resistance. The resistance can come in the form of weights, gravity, water, or even another part of your own body. Strengthening exercises help your muscles increase the force they can exert (strength) and the amount of time that they can exert it (endurance). Weight lifting, leg lifts, push-ups, swimming, and isometric exercises (e.g., placing your palms together and pushing them against each other) are all examples of strengthening exercises.
4. **Stretching**—These exercises increase your flexibility, and your ability to bend, twist, and reach. They increase the elasticity of your muscles; extend the range of motion of your joints; and make your muscles, tendons, ligaments, and joints more resistant to injury. They also relieve stress, ease muscle pain, and help you to relax. The best kind of stretching is called static stretching. You get into the stretching position and hold it at your maximum stretch for 30 to 45 sec-

onds. No bouncing (quickly pulling and releasing within the stretch) allowed! Toward the end of the 30 to 45 seconds, try to ease a little further into the stretch, hold it, and then slowly release. There are loads of great stretches for the neck, arms, sides, back, back of the legs, calves, and even the feet. Learn to stretch under the guidance of a trained professional, because you can do it incorrectly, and that can actually be worse than not stretching at all!

5. **Cooldown**—This is the flip side of the warm-up exercises, and often you can do the very same thing. The idea is to keep moving but to decelerate so that your body gets used to the idea that it's coming in for a landing.

PUTTING IT ALL TOGETHER

Now that you know the five elements of a good exercise program, here's how you put them together to create your own individualized fitness plan:

- Do your warm-up for 10 to 15 minutes at the beginning of your session. It doesn't matter what it is, as long as it gets your heart beating harder and your breath coming faster, without being overly strenuous. Ideally, you won't move on to the rest of your exercise program until you've broken a sweat.
- Cardiovascular-endurance exercises should be done for 20 consecutive minutes, 3 times a week. If you can't manage 30 minutes in the beginning, try 10 or even 5, just get started. In time, you'll be able to increase the length of your workouts. Your goal should be 30 minutes per session, 3 times a week.
- Strengthening exercises should be done on the days you don't do cardio exercises (e.g., cardio on Monday, Wednesday, Friday; strengthening on Tuesday, Thursday, Saturday). Begin with 10- to 15-minute sessions; build up to 20 to 30 minutes. Work carefully so you don't

strain or injure yourself. Ask your health advisor to help you devise a program.

- Stretching should be done every day for 15 to 20 minutes. You probably won't have time to stretch every area of your body in just 20 minutes, so do some overall stretches, then concentrate on a different area of your body each day (e.g., back stretches today, leg stretches tomorrow). Stretching is best done at the end of the workout, when you're thoroughly warmed up. Do not start your workout with stretches—your muscles aren't warm enough and you could injure yourself.
- Be sure to cool down—don't exercise at full capacity and then just stop dead! Take 5 to 10 minutes to ease yourself down to more sedentary levels by walking slowly, stretching, and taking some deep breathes.

THE BEST KIND OF EXERCISE

The best kind of exercise is whatever kind you'll actually do regularly. Find something you really like—something you love, if possible!—and make it an integral part of your life. Your health will bloom, and potentially, your asthma and allergies will wither.

9

Cut Back on Stress

Once, when I was visiting Rome, I had just stepped off the curb to cross the street when a speeding taxi flew around the corner and just about creamed me. Luckily, I saw something flying toward me and I jumped back on the sidewalk before I got hit. I was left gasping for breath, sweating, and weak in the knees, with my heart pounding in my ears—all the classic signs of stress—but I was okay. The good news is that your body's response to a potentially deadly situation can save your life. The bad news is that most of us experience the very same response several times a day when we're faced with things that are far from deadly: going on a date, getting cut off in traffic, or realizing that there's not much money left in the bank account. And over time, these stressors and your body's responses to them can wear down your resistance and contribute to a host of diseases and conditions, including allergies, asthma, eczema, hives, and psoriasis. While stress doesn't actually cause any of these, it can certainly make them worse. And once the symptoms set in, the fear and panic they cause can, in turn, become huge stressors that increase the reaction further.

One of the best things you can do for yourself is to promote a sense of calm and well-being. Relaxing, meditating, centering yourself, and refusing to get riled up over little things can do a lot to reduce both the frequency and intensity of your asthma and allergic reactions. In other words, learn to control stress or it will control you!

Handling the stress problem requires a two-pronged approach: first, you've got to reduce the level of stress in your life; second, you've got to learn to manage the stress that you can't get rid of.

REDUCING STRESS

A lot of our stress is self-induced. We want too much too soon and rush out into the world determined to get it. Then roadblocks crop up, and we become frustrated and stressed out. But, if we can induce our own stress, we can also reduce it. Consider these tips:

- **Slow down!** Take life a little slower. Stroll instead of hustle, talk more slowly, give the other person time to answer, and let their answers sink in before you rush to reply. Adopt the art of good conversation—that means really listening, not just using others as your audience.
- **Manage your time.** Prioritize your tasks and schedule them during your hours of peak efficiency. Budget a realistic amount of time to complete your tasks, then add a little more to allow for unforeseen circumstances. Get up earlier so you don't have to rush through your morning routine. Leave for work or school earlier than necessary, so traffic won't be such a stressor.
- **Set reasonable goals.** Determine what your goals are and then break them up into smaller goals that are more easily attainable. Don't overload yourself by trying to do too much too quickly or frustrate yourself by focusing only on long-term goals that obscure the slow-but-steady progress you're making on a daily basis.
- **Don't expect yourself to be perfect.** Nobody is. Enough said.
- **Don't expect perfection from others.** You're just going to be disappointed.

- **Learn to say "no."** Take on fewer projects. You don't have to do everything; just do a few things well.
- **Ask for help.** When you're feeling overwhelmed, ask for help from family members, friends, coworkers, or others in your support system. Hire help if you can—why should you have to clean the house if you're working full-time *and* raising a family?
- **Enjoy what you've got.** Do you have a good job, a nice family, a cozy home, a pretty garden? Good friends? Affectionate pets? Focus on the things in your life that are good and forget about the things that are bad. Just doing this should reduce your stress levels considerably.
- **Get plenty of sleep.** It will restore you.
- **Exercise.** Researchers have found that people who get regular exercise have milder physical responses to stressors and feel less hassled than those who don't exercise regularly. Even a brisk ten-minute walk can help relax and revive you. (See Chapter 8 for more on exercise.)
- **Adopt a hobby.** Make sure it's not related to business and you're not doing it for money. Just do it for fun!
- **Accept the things you can't change.**
- **Take breaks.** Little breaks during the day, weekends away, vacations to somewhere relaxing—all of these can work wonders. Enjoy yourself, because that's what life is all about!

RELAXATION TECHNIQUES

The opposite of stress is relaxation, when your body and mind enter a quiet, restful state while remaining awake and mentally alert. During relaxation your breathing, heart rate, metabolism, blood pressure, and consumption of oxygen all decline. In the brain, the alert beta waves become relaxed alpha waves. The best way to manage stress and its debilitating effects is to summon the relaxation response at least a couple of times a day, if possible. You can do this by using different relaxation techniques like meditation, progressive relaxation, and guided imagery.

Meditation

Meditation is a way to get your mind and your body to be quiet for a while. You can do this by focusing on a word, a phrase, or an object outside of yourself. When you assume a comfortable position in a quiet, peaceful environment and concentrate on this word, phrase, or object, the mind becomes more still, and relaxation will follow. Thoughts and images may drift in and out of your mind, but just ignore them and continue to concentrate. With practice, the relaxation response will become automatic whenever you sit quietly for a few minutes.

Programmed Relaxation

Another form of meditation is called programmed relaxation. With this technique, you focus on your muscles, tensing and relaxing them in a programmed manner. You might begin by tightening the muscles in your feet, holding the contraction for a count of 10, then relaxing your feet completely. Next contract your calves, hold, and then relax, working your way all the way up your body to your facial muscles. By contracting and releasing your muscles from stem to stern, you should be able to achieve a state of deep relaxation. Eventually, you may be able to reach this state of relaxation just by clenching and relaxing your fists.

Guided Imagery

Guided imagery is a way of putting yourself in a better place by imagining yourself in relaxing, beautiful, or otherwise desirable scenarios.

For example, you might imagine yourself relaxing in a hammock strung between two palm trees in Bora Bora, when you're actually stuffed into a crowded, smelly underground train. By doing so, you will be able to stay serene and happy, while everyone else is ready to tear their hair out.

This technique is often used by hypnotherapists and can be administered effectively via audiotapes. It's valuable not only as a relaxation tool but also as a way to visualize yourself achieving any goal—including fewer and milder symptoms of asthma or allergies and better health in general. It's a great way to relax while in the throes of an attack, thus helping ensure that stress doesn't make your condition worse.

Biofeedback

Biofeedback is a wonderful tool that can help you learn how to perform relaxation techniques more effectively. By showing you what's going on inside your body, both before and after relaxing, you'll learn which techniques work best for you and what you can do to increase their effectiveness. During biofeedback sessions, you'll be hooked up to electrical equipment that tracks your heart rate, blood pressure, muscle tension, temperature, and so forth. You'll be able to see how these rates change as you use relaxation and visualization techniques, and, with time, you may learn how to alter these bodily functions at will.

OTHER STRESS BUSTERS

These techniques are quick but powerful ways to defuse stress that can leave you feeling better immediately. Don't forget them in your quest to melt away the stressors in your life.

Breathing Exercises

Deep breathing is a fast and easy way to calm and energize your body all at once. Remember to breathe with your diaphragm (not your chest), fill the lungs completely, hold for a few counts, and then slowly exhale. After a few deep breaths you should already feel a marked reduction in stress. (See Chapter 7 for more on breathing.)

Laughter

A good belly laugh can actually reduce the levels of certain stress hormones in the blood. At the same time, your blood pressure and heart rate will also decrease. And after a good laugh, the problem (whatever it was) usually won't seem so overwhelming. So hang on to your sense of humor and realize that few things are really worth stewing about. Laugh it off, whenever possible!

Prayer

Communicating with a higher power is often a great antidote to stress. When things get too tough for us to handle all by ourselves, it's a great relief to hand them over to one who is greater than ourselves. Pray for strength, peace, health, the ability to conquer problems, or whatever else you need. This simple act can relieve stress, calm you, and bring miracles into your life. It works.

10

Think Positively

"I'm going to be sick; I know it, I just know it. My nose is going to run like Niagara Falls, and my eyes are going to water for forty days and forty nights."

Ever had such pleasant little thoughts? When you feel that little bit of scratchiness in your throat that just may herald the arrival of an asthma or allergy attack, do you automatically imagine the horrors that the next week or two might hold? Do you get an unshakeable feeling of dread when the first flowers begin to bloom or a cat walks into the room? Does your heart pound and your stomach start to ache as you wait for your skin to break out in a lovely, bright red rash?

If so, you're not alone. And, unfortunately, those thoughts are not alone either. Odd as it may seem, every thought that crosses our minds is accompanied by a corresponding change in body chemistry. Happy or positive thoughts actually produce helpful changes in the body while anxious, fearful, sad, or negative thoughts do just the opposite. Asthma, in particular, is linked to negative emotions such as fear or anxiety. In fact, the severity of an asthma attack is often directly related to how fearful, anxious, or angry a person is at the time.

Researchers at UCLA performed an interesting study on the effects of positive and negative emotions on the immune system. They had a group of method actors act out both happy and sad scenes. Before and after, the scientists checked the actors' saliva for certain antibodies that indicate the strength of the immune system. When the actors played out the happy scenes, the level of these antibodies increased, indicating that their immune systems were stronger. But, the sad scenes brought about the reverse reaction—decreased levels of antibodies, suggesting decreased immune activity. And that was just the result of acting, not living. If pretending to feel a certain way can quickly and obviously affect the immune system, just imagine what happens when you're really upset, depressed, angry, or stressed. Or, when you start telling yourself that you're about to suffer from a full-blown allergic reaction any day, hour, or minute, and it's going to be a doozy?

The UCLA-actors study isn't the only one that has shown a link between thoughts and the immune system or thoughts and physical health. Other studies have shown that:

- You can increase the activity of natural killer cells in your body and raise the levels of two heavyweight immune system "soldiers" (IgA and plasma cytokine gamma interferon) just by laughing.
- Stress increases both allergic and asthmatic responses.
- Positive thinking can increase the level of endorphins in the bloodstream. Endorphins are your body's natural painkilling, feel-good hormones.
- Stress, anger, and depression can alter your perception of pain, making you feel worse than you otherwise would.

WORDS CAN BECOME REALITY

One of the earliest observations of the strong link between thoughts and health came during World War II, thanks to a Western Union messenger named "Doc" Wiley. Doc was a happy guy who carried a pocketful of little slips of paper, on which he'd written slogans like,

"Today is a great day!" or "Pack up your troubles!" Each time he delivered a message for Western Union, he also gave out one of his slogans.

When the United States entered World War II, Doc volunteered to help out in a hospital. He emptied bedpans, helped soldiers get into and out of bed, and did whatever else he could to comfort them. Doc was happy to help in the war effort, but it was tough on him. He got very upset every time he had to wheel another dead soldier out of the ward. Doc didn't want anyone else to die, but he had no idea how to keep the wounded and sick men alive. After all, he wasn't a doctor. Then he thought about his slogans.

One morning, when the soldiers woke up, they were greeted by a huge message that had been painted on the walls of their ward. It read: "No one dies on this ward!" Of course, the folks who ran the hospital were furious about this vandalism, until one doctor spoke up. "Look!" he exclaimed. "The patients are laughing about what's been painted on the wall! They're making bets on who's going to last the longest. They're having fun and they look a lot healthier. Let's just leave the painted message alone and see what happens."

So they did, and the oddest thing happened: The soldiers stopped dying. They took Doc Wiley's exhortation to heart, and, somehow, it managed to change the chemistry of their bodies. It actually made them healthier. The patients on Doc Wiley's ward, the ones who read that positive message on the wall day after day, did better than those on the other wards. Of course, someone on Doc Wiley's ward did die eventually. But the other patients continued the trend of better health through positive thinking, thanks to Doc's message.

Back then, no one knew why Doc's message had such a positive effect. Doctors of that era didn't know much about the immune system and certainly didn't understand that it was connected to the nervous system and that messages could pass from the mind to the body. They didn't know, as we do today, that positive thoughts invariably tweak body chemistry for the better, and negative thoughts do the opposite.

Don't get me wrong, no one is claiming that your allergies will suddenly vanish if you simply click your heels together three times and say "I wish I were healthy, I wish I were healthy, I wish I were healthy." It is clear, however, that keeping a positive attitude will help your body remain as strong as it possibly can. And that alone may aid you in your quest to heal yourself—or at least to decrease your symptoms.

YOU *CAN* CHANGE YOUR THOUGHTS

How do you keep smiling when a skin rash makes you want to scratch your flesh off? How do you laugh when a runny nose makes you wish you had a faucet in your head that you could turn on full blast to get rid of the mucus all at once? You can start by realizing that the way you think about an event or a stressor will influence your feelings and behaviors (both inward and outward). When you first notice the event or stressor (e.g., some shortness of breath), slow down your thought processes and relax for a few moments. You have control of how you want to think about it. Instead of saying to yourself, "Oh no, here comes another asthma attack!" say, "I can handle this. I'm going to slow down now, take some deep breaths, and visualize the opening and relaxing of my bronchial tubes." Remember to keep the stressor or event in perspective, and make plans for the best way to handle the situation.

Besides taking control of your thoughts, try laughing more (unless this happens to be an asthma trigger for you). Did you know that the average child laughs some four hundred times a day, while we grown-ups laugh a measly six to eight times? Increasing your laugh-per-minute ratio is a great way to put yourself in a positive frame of mind. Allow yourself to laugh more, and look for opportunities to do so. Read joke books, see funny movies, and watch silly sitcoms. Ask people if they have any good jokes to tell you. If your friends send you jokes and comics via the Internet, print them out, and save them for future tickling of the funny bone. Stand out on the lawn in your bathing suit with your arms spread and the sprinklers going full blast. Participate in fun events like Halloween parties or sing-a-longs. Or start the "dress-like-your-favorite-character-from-'Star Trek' day" at work. Live a little; it will increase your positivity quotient!

Here are some other ways to generate positive thoughts and feel good about yourself:

- Volunteer at a senior citizens center.
- Participate in a wilderness cleanup project.
- Help serve meals to the homeless.
- Mentor a disadvantaged youngster.
- Play with your kids.
- Visit a beautiful garden.
- Create your own beautiful garden.
- Exercise.
- Meditate.
- Read something uplifting.
- Call your mother.
- Make something by hand.
- Count your blessings.

Finally, adopt a positive philosophy about life. Instead of wondering if the glass is half full or half empty, just grab that glass and start drinking! Positive thinking won't magically eliminate your asthma or allergy symptoms, but it will help ease the way and make everything seem a little (or a lot) better.

11

Help Yourself with Hypnosis

When I was in my early twenties, I went to see a show put on by a locally famous hypnotist who used his skills for entertainment purposes. When he asked for volunteers, my hand shot up, and before I knew it I was one of ten subjects up on stage. He put us under, then asked us to imagine that our arms were weightless and floating away, and, sure enough, our arms started rising up and waving in the breeze. He went through several other similar stunts before he asked, "Who came with a date tonight?" Once again my hand shot up, along with those of a few of my cohorts. My date, a guy I barely knew and had never been out with before, was sitting in the audience watching my antics with what I can only imagine was amused disbelief. "Okay," said the hypnotist, "The next time you hear me say the word 'rabbit,' I want you to run out into the audience, grab your date, and start kissing him. And I don't want you to stop until I say 'green grass.'"

A feeling of pure dread crept through my body. Kiss him? We hadn't even held hands yet! And besides, I wasn't sure how well I liked him. After a few more hypnotic stunts, the hypnotist suddenly said the word "rabbit." And it was as if my feet had a will of their own. Looking down, I could see my brown sandals hightailing it out into the audience in search of you-know-who. And there we stood, passionately making out in front of about two hundred people for what seemed like an eternity, until we finally heard the words "green grass."

I bring this up now only because I truly believe that my behavior that night was due to the power of hypnosis. The hypnotist planted a suggestion in my mind, and my body seemed hell-bent on carrying it out. And if we can use that power for entertainment purposes, we certainly ought to be able to put it to work curing our ills and fortifying our health.

I have to admit that I'm not the first person to make this brilliant deduction. Back in the 1770s, Dr. Franz Anton Mesmer was able to relieve pain and treat illness mostly through the power of his soothing and persuasive personality—he *mesmerized* his patients. Psychotherapists have long used hypnosis to help their patients change attitudes or behaviors. And hypnosis has gained great popularity in recent years as a way to help people lose weight, overcome addictions, lessen pain, reduce fatigue, ease anxiety and depression, or get rid of bad habits. Plus, the medical community now considers hypnosis to be an effective form of treatment for stress-related conditions like migraines, hypertension, and irritable bowel syndrome. So if stress, negative thoughts, anger, frustration, and general upsets can make your asthma and allergies worse, it's not hard to see that hypnosis, with its calming, relaxing influence, can also help calm your body and its hypersensitive reactions.

In spite of the fact that hypnosis is sometimes used for entertainment, it's really not a trick. Instead, it's a way to alter your consciousness, bring about relaxation, focus your attention, and make it easier for you to use techniques like positive thinking, visualization, guided imagery, and stress release. In the process, hypnosis can help you stop an asthma attack in its early stages, reduce allergic symptoms, and possibly even reduce the amount of medication you require.

HOW HYPNOSIS WORKS

You'll probably be able to hypnotize yourself eventually, but first you'll need to see a professional hypnotist so you can learn the ropes. The hypnotist will take a history, find out what problems you'd like addressed, and so forth, and then ask you to sit in a comfortable chair, close your eyes, and relax. She will probably suggest that you are becoming sleepy or your eyes are heavy and invite you to give in to that feeling. Then some sort of visual picture will be suggested. You may be asked to visualize a long flight of stairs, for example, and as you descend those stairs, you'll ease deeper and deeper into the relaxed feeling or trance.

Once you are completely relaxed and your mind is open to suggestion, the hypnotist will paint a different picture with words, calling up the problem you're experiencing. If it's asthma, for example, you may be asked to visualize something like this:

> Imagine yourself standing on top of a mountain with pure, sweet, fresh air all around you. Visualize your breathing tubes as wide open, with air flowing freely in and out. As you draw in a breath, you find it's so easy to fill your lungs with pure, sweet air. Then it's even easier to exhale that air, all the way, down to the last molecule. It feels so good to breathe deeply and easily.

Then you'll be given a posthypnotic suggestion—that is, the planting of a certain thought or behavior that will automatically be triggered when a specific situation arises. For example, the hypnotist might say, "Whenever you begin to feel bronchial constriction, you'll automatically visualize this mountain top and see yourself taking slow, deep, invigorating breaths. Your bronchial tubes will relax and widen, letting the delicious air flow easily into and out of your lungs."

For allergies, the same basic technique can be used, but the visual picture and posthypnotic suggestion will be different. The hypnotist might say:

> As you're sitting here relaxing, in your mind's eye notice the rash on your arm. You can see that it's red, inflamed, and bumpy. It itches and maybe even burns a little. Now, imagine that you're holding a tube of cool, ice-blue healing lotion. You pour a little of that healing lotion into your hand and rub it gently on the rash. It feels so soothing, cooling, and calming. As you massage the cream into your skin, you notice that the rash has begun to fade. The more you stroke your skin, the more the rash recedes. And in its place you can see smooth, unbroken skin, glowing with health. Once you're done massaging your arm, notice that the rash has completely disappeared. Your skin feels and looks completely healed.

The posthypnotic suggestion might be that the next time you feel a rash coming on, you will instantly find a quiet place, sit down, relax, and think of the ice-blue healing cream soothing the rash away. This may not completely eradicate the rash, of course, but it will probably ease the intensity of the reaction.

FINDING A QUALIFIED HYPNOTHERAPIST

It's best to find a clinically trained hypnotherapist (a psychologist, doctor, or nurse) for maximum therapeutic benefits. To find one, contact the National Guild of Hypnotists at P.O. Box 308, Merrimack, New Hampshire 03054-0308; phone 603-429-9438; or visit their website, ngh.net.

12
Yoga

I first became acquainted with yoga back in the late 1960s when rock musicians and Hollywood starlets began making highly publicized sojourns to India to live in ashrams and learn the latest fad in the healing arts. Although it sounded like a brand-new, superhip idea to my teenage girlfriends and me, it was actually as old as the hills, dating as far back as 3000 B.C.

Yoga, a system of physical, mental, emotional, and spiritual development, gets its name from the Sanskrit word *yug*, which means "yoke" or "a joining together." Its aim is to join the body, mind, emotions, and spirit in a harmonious union. There are many different branches of yoga, but the one most often practiced here in North America is *raja*, a system that involves postures, deep breathing, and progressive relaxation. One of the primary aims of yoga is restoration of the *prana*, or life energy, the vital force that flows through the bodies of every living thing.

The special yoga postures or poses (called *asanas*) are great for increasing flexibility, releasing muscle tension, revving up circulation, toning muscles, and encouraging relaxation. The breathing exercises (called *pranayama*) expand the capacity of the lungs, improve respiration, and slow the breathing, while restoring the prana and keeping it moving freely throughout the body. And the progressive relaxation exercises relieve stress and muscle tension, improve immune system function, balance the nervous system, lower the blood pressure, and just generally make you feel great.

Yoga is a health-enhancer for just about anybody, but for those with asthma or allergies it can be a real boon. Because stress, nervous tension, and emotional upsets can increase or even cause asthmatic or allergic reactions, it makes sense that yoga, with its relaxing, stress-relieving effects, can be a big help in calming them down. The pranayama are particularly therapeutic for asthmatics. By encouraging slower, deeper, more controlled breathing, they increase lung capacity, strengthen the respiratory system as a whole, and help reduce both the frequency and severity of asthma attacks.

The postures are usually done slowly and are combined with the breathing: the pose is usually held for several counts while slowly inhaling, holding the breath for a few counts, then exhaling. (A few of the major breathing exercises can be found in Chapter 7.) The following are descriptions of some typical yoga postures. All are good for general relaxation and improving breathing capacity, and special areas targeted by the exercises are noted.

THE CHILD'S POSE

This exercise will increase spinal flexibility.

1. Sit with your legs tucked underneath you, knees pointing straight ahead, heels directly under your buttocks.
2. Separate your knees about 12 inches, but keep your big toes touching each other, each foot pointing slightly inward, toward the center of your body.
3. Extend your upper body forward toward the floor, arms extended, hands flat on the floor, forehead touching the floor if possible.

4. Try to keep your heels in contact with your buttocks as you hold this pose for a count of 20.
5. Slowly roll back to sitting position.

KNEE TO CHEST

This pose will increase the flexibility of the hip joints, buttock muscles, and lower back.

1. Lie on your back with arms at your sides and legs extended.
2. Inhale; bend your right leg and bring it toward your chest, holding just below the knee with both hands.
3. Pull your knee gently toward your chest as far as it will go. Hold it there for a count of 5, keeping the other leg straight and in contact with the floor.
4. Exhale slowly as you release.
5. Repeat with the opposite leg.

BODY TWIST

Practice this pose to increase the flexibility of the hips, spine, upper chest, and neck muscles.

1. Lie on your back, with your legs extended and arms at your sides.
2. As in the Knee to Chest exercise, inhale, bend your right leg, grab it just below the knee with both hands, and pull it gently toward your chest as far as it will go.
3. Use your left hand only to pull your right knee across your body toward the floor on your left side.
4. Meanwhile, extend your right arm to your right, perpendicular to your body. Press your right shoulder blade

to the floor while you press your knee toward the left. (You'll feel a good stretch in your spine.)

5. Turn your head toward your extended arm, exhale, and hold this position for a count of 15.
6. Repeat using your right hand and your left knee, with your left arm extended and head turned toward left.

THE PRETZEL

This pose will increase inner-thigh and hip flexibility.

1. Lie on your back with your arms at your sides and your knees bent.
2. Cross your left leg over your right, placing your left foot on your right thigh, just above the knee. The left knee should point straight to the side.
3. Slowly inhale, and using both hands, grab hold of your right thigh and slowly pull it toward you without uncrossing your legs.
4. Hold for at least 5 seconds.
5. Slowly exhale as you release, then repeat with the opposite leg.

THE CAT

This pose increases spinal flexibility.

1. As if you were a cat, get on all fours with your weight evenly distributed between your palms and knees. Fingers should point forward with your knees about 10 inches apart.

2. Slowly inhale as you tighten your stomach muscles and round your lower back toward the ceiling, forming a cave with your abdominal muscles.
3. At the same time, pull your chin toward your chest. Your entire spine should look like the top half of the letter "O." Hold for a count of 5.
4. Slowly exhale as you relax your spine; then begin to arch it backward slightly so that it resembles a slight smile.
5. At the same time, gradually ease your head backward until your chin is parallel to the floor.
6. Gradually go back to the starting position, and repeat, taking the spine through its range of movement without straining or forcing.

THE SNAKE

If you want to increase arm and upper-body strength and flexibility of the chest, stomach, and back muscles, practice this pose.

1. Lie face down on a mat with elbows bent and the palms of the hands resting on either side of the neck, parallel to the sides of the face.
2. Inhale slowly as you press the hands into the mat, and, using the lower arms, slowly raise the head and upper chest until they are completely off the floor. Don't bend the head back too far; keep the neck in line with the spine.
3. Gradually straighten the arms as you push the head, chest, and torso as far up as they'll go. (Keep the pelvis flat on the floor, with legs extended.)
4. Hold for a count of 5.

5. Exhale slowly as you bend the arms and ease the torso back down to the mat.
6. Return to starting position.

FINDING A QUALIFIED INSTRUCTOR

Make sure you learn the correct techniques from a qualified yoga instructor, at least in the beginning. Books or videotapes just don't cut it when you're still a novice, because they can't tell you what you're doing wrong. You'll need somebody with you, so he or she can make sure you're assuming the positions correctly. Otherwise, chances are good that you'll stretch the wrong muscles (or the right muscles in the wrong way) and end up doing more harm than good. Books and videotapes are fine, of course, once you're sure of the techniques.

To learn more about yoga and how to choose a good yoga instructor, contact the American Yoga Association, P.O. Box 19986, Sarasota, Florida 34276; phone 800-226-5859; or visit their website at http://members.aol.com/amyogaassn/index.htm, then click on Yoga Teachers.

13

Bolster Health with Bee Products

From the honey bee, one of the hardest working creatures on earth, we get the gift of three miraculous substances that can detoxify the body, stimulate the immune system, control weight, mitigate the ill effects of stress, quell anxiety, increase energy, and ease allergies. Does that sound improbable, coming from the same scary little insect that made your foot burn, itch, and swell like crazy last summer when you were walking barefoot in the backyard? Not according to proponents of bee pollen, bee propolis, and royal jelly.

BEE POLLEN

This nutritious substance is made of the pollen that's taken from flowering plants and is then mixed with honey. As bees flit from flower to flower, bits of live pollen (the male seed or fertilizer for flowers) cling to their legs. The bees mix this pollen with a little bit of honey and then carry it back to the hive. The resultant mixture, called *bee pollen*, contains a potpourri of vitamins, minerals, amino acids, fatty acids, protein, carbohydrates, lecithin, quercetin, lycopene, and other substances. Bee pollen is sometimes called nature's perfect food because it's believed to contain all of the necessary nutrients for human nutrition. Used to treat a variety of ailments, including the symptoms of certain allergies, a key attribute of bee pollen is its antihistamine effects. Oddly enough, the same little insect that can cause inflammation with its nasty sting can also produce an anti-inflammatory agent. For some people, regular ingestion of bee pollen reduces or completely relieves the symptoms of allergic rhinitis, pollen-induced asthma, or bronchitis.

Caution: bee pollen may trigger an allergic reaction in susceptible people.

BEE PROPOLIS

Bee propolis has been used as a healing agent for thousands of years. In fact, Hippocrates, the father of modern medicine, used propolis internally to heal ulcers and externally for wound healing. Also known as "bee glue," it's made from the sticky resin and ooze of certain trees, mixed with a substance secreted by the bee. Bees use propolis as a structural material to plug up holes in their hives, seal off dead matter that's too large to remove, and line every bit of the inside of the hive to keep it germ-free. When spread out and allowed to dry, it forms a tough, hard surface. (It's been said that Antonio Stradivari mixed bee propolis into the varnishes he applied to his famous violins.)

Because propolis has strong antibacterial and antifungal properties, it's sometimes referred to as nature's penicillin. It's also rich in vitamins, bioflavonoids, and other health-enhancing substances and may be able to help fight infections, ease eczema and skin rashes, reduce allergy symptoms, and promote healthy immune function. Skin irritations may also be calmed through the use of bee propolis cream.

Caution: Bee propolis contains bee pollen and may trigger an allergic reaction.

ROYAL JELLY

Talk about fit for a queen! This nutrient-rich substance is specially made by bees solely for feeding the queen bee (always) and the worker bees (during the first three days of their lives). Manufactured in the bodies of nurse bees who have eaten bee pollen, royal jelly contains loads of protein, vitamins, amino acids, fatty acids, DNA, RNA, natural hormones, and other superduper health enhancers.

Royal jelly contains vitamins A, C, D, E, and B-complex vitamins (including plenty of pantothenic acid, which is believed to strengthen the adrenal glands and help reduce stress). It also contains six minerals (sodium, potassium, iron, chromium, manganese, and nickel) and various amino acids. Royal jelly has both antibiotic and antibacterial effects, fighting the growth of bacteria that cause skin or intestinal infections. It can also reestablish the acid mantle of the skin, helping to fight skin ailments.

In short, royal jelly can bolster your vitamin and mineral intake, fight infections, and ease allergic skin reactions. It can also speed the healing process and ease the symptoms of stress.

DO BEE PRODUCTS WORK?

The idea that the busy little bees can make medicine for man is not a new one. Ancient Egyptian doctors considered honey to be a universal healer, and the Chinese used it to treat smallpox and other ailments. More recently, American and British researchers have shown that raw honey helps heal wounds and can also destroy bacteria. Many feel that the ingredient in raw honey that's responsible for its medicinal success is bee pollen.

Today, many proponents of alternative healing praise bee pollen, bee propolis, and royal jelly for their ability to detoxify the body, stimulate the immune system, improve strength and endurance, help regulate blood pressure, treat prostate infections, heighten mental alertness, and help relieve allergy symptoms.

As of yet, there isn't a large body of scientific research to back up these claims, so we have to rely largely on anecdotal evidence—and there is a fair amount of that. Both doctors and patients have reported that many of the symptoms of several types of allergies, including hay fever, are relieved by the regular ingestion of bee pollen (as opposed to taking it only when symptoms strike). The number of allergy attacks drops, sometimes dramatically, and the remaining attacks are much less severe. Some people report that their allergy problems disappear almost entirely.

How does it work? We don't really know. The three bee products contain significant amounts of nutrients and other substances that strengthen the immune system and possibly help regulate certain body activities. In this way, bee pollen, bee propolis, and royal jelly may improve the body's ability to heal itself. Bee pollen may also reduce the body's production of histamine, which could explain why bee products have anti-allergy effects. It may also be that bee products supply the nutrients the body needs to fight disease or maintain homeostasis.

BUYING BEE POLLEN

Bee products are not subject to the same stringent processing, packaging, shipping, and storage requirements that govern drugs, so there are definite variations in quality from product to product. Make sure you buy from reliable sources, and look for pollen that's a standardized blend from a variety of different geographic locations. This will help ensure that the pollen has all the necessary ingredients. If you can find out about how the pollen was processed, look for a brand that was deep-frozen immediately after it was collected, then kept dry and frozen until packaging. Beware of pollen that has been heat-treated, because this can destroy some of the nutrients.

TAKING BEE PRODUCTS

The use of bee products is an inexact science, because optimal doses have not yet been determined. In other words, we just don't know how much you should take. The best idea is to work with your physician to see if the "three bees" can help combat your allergies. Start slowly, with minimal doses, since some allergic reactions are possible. (Although ingesting bee pollen in pill form is not the same as inhaling pollen that's floating in the air, it's best to be cautious until you're sure that you won't get a reaction.)

To find out more about bee pollen or products, contact the C. C. Pollen Company at 3627 E. Indian School Road, Suite 209, Phoenix, Arizona 85018-5126; phone 602-957-0096; or visit their website, ccpollen.com.

14

Adjust Your Health with Chiropractic and Osteopathy

Back in the 1870s, an American physician named Andrew Still was crushed when his wife and three of their children came down with meningitis and eventually died. Determined to succeed where standard Western medicine had failed, he thought long and hard about the possible causes of all diseases and their cures. Still believed that man was created in God's image and that the human body was an earthly symbol of God's perfection. Thus, a body in its pristine state simply couldn't be diseased. To this basic premise he added the observation that nerve impulses and fluids continuously move through the body, but that during illness their normal flow is disrupted. Tying it all together, Still concluded that disease must be caused by a disruption of the normal flow of nerve impulses and fluids throughout the body. From these principles came the practice of osteopathy, which teaches that the body can't function properly unless it's structurally sound, and that the cure for disease lies in manipulating the body's tissues and joints to restore the normal flow of fluid and nerve impulses.

Some twenty years later, a Canadian man named David Palmer came to a similar conclusion, but his ideas focused entirely on the spine. Palmer argued that disease began when nerves running along the spine were pinched, pressed, or otherwise interfered with by the spinal vertebrae. When that happened, the parts of the body serviced by that nerve became damaged, thus setting the stage for disease.

These two therapies—osteopathy and chiropractic—struggled for decades under the suspicious and skeptical eyes of Western medical doctors. But thirty or forty years ago, osteopathy more or less merged with standard Western medicine, and today a doctor of osteopathy (DO) is legally the same as a medical doctor (MD). DOs study at four-year medical colleges, go through a residency, practice medicine and surgery, and can become board certified in a specialty. In fact, the former U.S. Surgeon General Dr. C. Everett Koop is not an MD but a DO. The only difference between an MD and a DO these days is that the osteopaths take a few courses in the manipulation techniques that were originated by Dr. Still.

Chiropractic has not fared quite as well. Through the 1960s, physicians who worked with chiropractors, or even associated with them personally, were considered unethical and at risk of censure by their local medical associations. But in recent years, the medical profession has seen the light as far as the value of chiropractic adjustments for certain conditions, and today many physicians refer their patients to chiropractors. As a final stamp of approval, chiropractic is now covered by many insurance plans.

CHIROPRACTIC TECHNIQUE

Chiropractors used to be thought of as nothing more than "back crackers," but there's a lot more to this healing art than that. The heart of chiropractic theory involves the *subluxation*, the pressing of the spinal vertebrae on nerves. Subluxations can be caused by all kinds of things, including injury, bad posture, stress, poor lifting habits, lack of exercise, and genetic imbalances. Most of the time, subluxations are not painful in and of themselves, so we probably don't even realize that there's a problem. Instead, we focus on the symptoms caused by the subluxation, like a neck ache or tight shoulder muscles. We're not very likely to associate a migraine headache, for example, with a slight spinal misalignment, although that could be the cause.

So, if subluxations are the cause of a disease, the solution, it seems, would be to move those errant bones around until they stop pinching on your nerves. And that's exactly what doctors of chiropractic try to do. To diagnose and treat spinal misalignments, a chiropractor will ask you about your symptoms, the diseases you've had, the accidents you've suffered, your exercise and lifestyle habits, and so forth. He will also observe the way you stand and use your body and may take an x-ray of the affected part.

Then the chiropractor will get to work with his main tool: his hands. While you lie on a padded table, he will feel along your spine, trying to find the vertebrae that are out of alignment, as well as any swelling, muscle tension, or other signs of spinal distress. Once the problem has been discovered, he will use various hands-on techniques to realign the spine, by pushing, pulling, massaging, and pressing on muscles, joints, and connective tissue. This process is known as an *adjustment*.

Today, there are two general types of chiropractors. First there are those who limit themselves to manipulating the spine in order to cure subluxations. The second type includes those who manipulate the spine and borrow from a variety of other therapies, including homeopathy, nutrition, and other forms of bodywork to help solve the problem and get your body back into shape.

OSTEOPATHIC TECHNIQUE

Osteopathy is somewhat similar to chiropractic but more complex. According to the American Osteopathic Association, osteopathy combines modern medical techniques with the understanding of "the interrelationship of structure and function, as well as the body's ability to heal itself." In other words, they use the same regular medical techniques as MDs (drugs and surgery) and then go beyond to include bodywork and manipulation of the spine, joints, and soft tissues. They call what they do *articulatory techniques*. They also use muscle energy manipulation, myofascial tissue release, and other bodywork techniques, including cranial osteopathy. Because they are licensed medical doctors, they can also prescribe medication for your asthma or allergies, when necessary.

Developed in the 1950s, cranial osteopathy is based on the idea that the cerebrospinal fluid moves in rhythmic pulses, and that disturbances in the flow can lead to physical and emotional ailments. By gently manipulating the bones of the head, the doctor attempts to restore the natural rhythm of the flow.

HOW CHIROPRACTIC AND OSTEOPATHY CAN HELP

While neither technique combats allergies directly, both osteopathy and chiropractic attempt to realign the body so that it can heal itself. Both kinds of manipulation may be able to help ease your asthma by working on your upper body to open up your chest, improve your posture, and otherwise make it easier for you to breathe, while improving your overall sense of well-being. Some chiropractors also believe that asthma may have something to do with a misalignment of the upper or center part of the spine, and that adjustments in these areas can ease asthmatic symptoms.

Be cautious, however. Theoretically, any pushing, pulling, twisting, or pressing on the bones or joints can be dangerous. Although the vast majority of people who undergo chiropractic or osteopathic manipulation suffer no ill effects, you should be aware of the possibilities.

FINDING A QUALIFIED PRACTITIONER

If you're going to let somebody rearrange something as important as your spine, you'd better find someone who really knows what he or she is doing. For a list of qualified chiropractors in your area, contact the American Chiropractic Association (ACA) at 1701 Clarendon Boulevard, Arlington, Virginia 22209; phone 800-986-4636; or visit their website, amerchiro.org. To find a doctor of osteopathy, contact the American Academy of Osteopathy at 3500 Depauw Boulevard, Suite 1080, Indianapolis, Indiana 46268-1136; phone 317-879-1881; or visit their website, academyofosteopathy.org.

15

Marvelous Massage

Massage, the "laying on of hands," has always been high on my list of wonderfully relaxing, restorative, and therapeutic treatments. We all need physical contact with another human being, but massage elevates touching to a high art and a healing one, at that. Our word *massage* comes from the Arabic word *massa*, which means "to stroke," and refers to the hands-on rubbing, kneading, or stroking of the skin and the application of pressure to the skin and muscles that lie beneath it. A good massage can do a lot more than just make you feel great, which in itself is no small thing. It can also do any or all of the following.

- Calm your nerves
- Ease tension
- Greatly increase overall relaxation
- Stimulate circulation
- Increase your endorphin levels, producing a wonderful natural "high"
- Loosen your muscles
- Melt away mental stress
- Ease pain by clearing away some of the irritating by-products of muscle metabolism

- Slow your heart rate
- Promote harmony in both mind and body
- Ease asthma symptoms by loosening up chest and back muscles

Because massage is a terrific stress reliever, it also helps bolster your immune system. When you're under stress, powerful chemicals, like cortisol, that can actually counteract immune function are released into your bloodstream. Your immune system, then, is already fighting an uphill battle before it's even begun to take on the enemy. Massage can help lower your levels of cortisol and other stress-related hormones, so your immune system can concentrate on fighting enemies from without rather than from within.

Massage also stimulates the circulation of the lymph, the fluid that carries waste and impurities away from the body. Unlike blood, which is propelled through the veins and arteries by the pumping of the heart, this milky-white fluid must be moved through the lymph system by the squeezing action of muscle contractions. Massage can mimic this squeezing action and help get the lymph moving so that waste and toxins are flushed out of the body faster.

TYPES OF MASSAGE

Although there are lots of different kinds of massage, these three techniques are found in most massage therapists' bag of tricks and are well worth investigating.

Swedish Massage

Also known as *effleurage*, this method of massage involves the kneading and stroking of the skin and muscles and the exertion of pressure on tense or knotted areas. Therapists often use oil or lotion to prevent friction and sometimes use aromatherapy (via scented oils, scented pillows, vaporizers, and so forth) to enhance the massage. Besides kneading and stroking, typical Swedish massage techniques include tapping or clapping movements, striking with cupped hands, squeezing or rolling the muscles, or chopping movements with the sides of the hands. (All of these methods feel a lot better than they sound!) Swedish massage can be done as gently or as vigorously as you like, with fast or slow stroking. Generally, the slower the strokes, the more relaxing, while faster strokes are more invigorating.

Shiatsu

Also known as acupressure, shiatsu is another form of massage that has gained great popularity in the United States in recent years. It's used to release energy blockages and restore the flow of the life force, or *chi*. (You'll find that many massage therapists like to use a combination of shiatsu and Swedish massage.) Shiatsu is a lot like acupuncture, but the fingers are used to stimulate the acupuncture points instead of needles. With fingers, hands, thumbs, elbows, feet, or special tools like wooden rollers, balls, or pointers, the practitioner applies pressure along specific energy channels, or *meridians*, to unblock the energy flow and restore balance to your body. In the process, the practitioner will also transmit some of his or her own energy to you. Results include relief from pain, renewed energy, and increased relaxation.

Trigger Point Therapy

Trigger point therapy involves the application of intense, prolonged pressure to specific points on painful, knotted muscles. I've had this done on my neck and upper back many times, and I won't mince words—it hurts! The therapist really digs his thumb into my knotted muscles and then presses as hard as he can for about thirty seconds. The idea is to overload the pain sensors in that area so they will stop sending pain messages back to the brain. It's literally a pain in the neck, but once the pressure is released, the ache generated by those knotted muscles vanishes as if by magic. If you have chronic tension that knots your muscles and causes pain, trigger point therapy may be the perfect solution.

MASSAGE FOR ALLERGIES AND ASTHMA

The biggest advantage that massage has to offer asthma and allergy sufferers is relief from stress. Stress, as we all know, makes everything worse, especially asthma or allergies. The accumulation of stress-related emotions like frustration, anxiety, or anger can themselves bring on asthma or allergy symptoms. By using massage to keep your stress levels in check, you may be able to reduce both the number and the severity of the attacks.

It's also been found that those with allergic rhinitis tend to carry extra tension in their chest and shoulder muscles. Massaging these areas helps promote relaxation and balance, which may help reduce hypersensitivity. At the very least, the easing of tension in these overly stressed areas should increase your feeling of well-being.

Finally, massage may help you loosen your chest and back muscles so that you can open up your chest cavity and breathe more deeply and easily. You've got to give your lungs room to expand if you want to get vital, nourishing oxygen into your body, and massage can help you do that.

MAXIMIZING THE HEALING EFFECTS OF MASSAGE

The basic idea behind massage is to help you relax deeply. But that can be difficult if you are not sure what to expect, you're worried about taking your clothes off in front of the therapist, you've rushed in five minutes late because of a traffic jam, or life in general has wound you tighter than your grandfather's watch. To really benefit from your massage, consider the following suggestions:

- Have a short chat with your therapist before the massage, letting her know about your health problems, any injuries or sore spots, the kind of massage you'd like, the results you're looking for, and so forth. Ask about the kinds of massage the therapist can perform, and request any that sound interesting.
- If possible, take a nice warm shower or bath right before your massage to get a head start on relaxation.
- If you're going to the therapist's office, leave early so traffic won't stress you or make you late. If the therapist is coming to you, be ready so you're not rushing around at the last minute.
- Don't eat or drink anything for at least thirty minutes before the session. (A gurgling stomach, acid reflux, or heartburn can detract from your relaxation.)
- If you feel funny about taking off your clothes, don't. Leave your underwear on, if you like, or wear even more than that. The most important thing is that you feel comfortable. (Of course, the best results are achieved when the massage therapist can make direct contact with your skin, so the less you wear the better, once you're comfortable with the idea.)
- If there are certain areas that you don't want massaged (for example, your feet), tell the therapist. (Breasts and genital areas are never massaged, so you won't have to worry about that.) It's up to you which areas of your body will be massaged. Your therapist should be happy to accommodate you.
- Communicate with your massage therapist during the massage. Tell him what hurts, what feels good, whether you'd like the pressure increased or decreased, and so forth. Everyone's different, and the therapist won't know what feels best to you unless you speak up.
- Take it easy once the massage is finished. Don't leap off the table, throw on your clothes, and zip off to do errands. Take a nap if pos-

sible, or just sit quietly. This is a great time for practicing deep breathing techniques.

- Always drink plenty of water after your massage is finished to help flush out circulating toxins.

FINDING A QUALIFIED MASSAGE THERAPIST

For a list of qualified massage therapists and the kinds of massage they offer, contact the American Massage Therapy Association at 820 Davis Street, Suite 100, Evanston, Illinois 60201; phone 847-864-0123; or visit their website, amtamassage.org. You can also contact the National Certification Board for Therapeutic Massage and Bodywork at 8301 Greensboro Drive, Suite 300, McLean, Virginia 22102; phone 800-296-0664; or visit their website, ncbtmb.com.

Many massage therapists do shiatsu, but if you'd like a list of certified acupressurists, you can get one from the National Certification Commission for Acupuncture and Oriental Medicine (NCCAOM) at 11 Canal Center Plaza, Suite 330, Alexandria, Virginia 22314; phone 703-548-9004; or visit their website, nccaom.org.

16

Pinpoint the Problem with Korean Hand Therapy

Last fall I managed to drag my husband Jack along with me to a medical convention. (I like to think he went along just because he loves spending time with me, but the truth is he only went because it was in Las Vegas.) While there, we both became fascinated by a new therapy from Korea that was presented at the convention and was touted as a way to relieve asthma and allergy symptoms, among other things. After the lecture, I managed to set up an interview with the speaker, and, naturally, I brought Jack along as my "demonstration dummy."

The approach, called Korean hand therapy (also known as Koryo hand therapy, or KHT), was developed by a doctor of Oriental medicine named Tae-Woo Yoo. Dr. Yoo had often been kept awake by headaches until he realized that by pressing certain points on his hands he could relieve the pain and get a decent night's sleep. That led him to the discovery that specific points on the hands correspond to various parts of the body, and that the application of pressure and other forms of stimulation to those points could help relieve pain.

BALANCING THE BLOOD FLOW

Of course, it's a bit more complex than that. It begins—and ends—with the idea that we need a balanced flow of blood to the brain in order to remain healthy. An imbalance reflects disease-related pain. This balance is assessed by a unique *yin* and *yang* pulse-testing method. The essential goal of KHT is to restore and maintain health by balancing the blood flow to the brain, which is done by manipulating specific points on the fronts or backs of the hands. Simply put, the idea is that pressing point A might relieve pain or other adverse reactions in point B by balancing the pulse and improving the flow of blood to the brain.

I was eager to try it, but I didn't have any pain or other body troubles on that particular day. (Lucky me!) My dear Jack, however, was suffering from a mild asthma attack that day, so (after much coaxing) I got him to sit down with the KHT practitioner, Dan Lobash, Ph.D., L.Ac. We deliberately didn't tell him anything about Jack's condition. Dr. Lobash felt Jack's carotid pulse (in the neck) and radial pulse (in the wrist). He told us that they were out of balance and one was thicker (meaning it had more blood flow) than the other.

The diagnosis of the cause of the imbalance was arrived at by exploring Jack's hands with a blunt-tipped metal probe about the size of a pen. As Dr. Lobash poked and prodded Jack's hands, he explained that the hand is a map of the body and that every part of the body has a corresponding point on the hand. The points for the head, for example, are found along the tips of each middle finger, those for the throat a little below on the palm side of the same finger, and those for the chest and heart are still lower.

The general map is easy to follow. The front of the hand (palm side) corresponds to the front of the body, the back of the hand to the back of the body. The front of the middle finger, starting at the top and moving down joint by joint, represents the head, neck, and chest. The index and ring fingers correspond to the left and right hands and arms, the thumb and pinkie to the feet and legs. The palm of the hand corresponds to the abdominal region; the back of the palm corresponds to the area from about the midback down to the bottom of the buttocks. There's a lot more to it than that, but you get the general idea.

That's the easy part. It gets a little confusing when you overlay a second map onto the first one. This second map is based on the concept of energy pathways on the fingers and hands (meridians) used for the flow of bio-energy, or *chi*, as it's called in traditional Chinese medicine. Rather than going into confusing detail, let's just say that the numerous points on the second map of the hands give the KHT therapist additional ways to treat your ailment, as well as your entire body.

Slowly and methodically, Dr. Lobash pushed his probe firmly into various points on Jack's hand, and Jack didn't bat an eye or respond in any way at first. But when the doctor put his probe on the chest point (which is on the front side of the middle finger), Jack's eyes suddenly opened wide and his back stiffened.

"Yeeouch!" he exclaimed.

"Ah, I see you're having problems with your chest," the doctor said.

"Yes," Jack said through clenched teeth. "And now my finger hurts, too."

Dr. Lobash probed the corresponding point on Jack's other hand and got an equally enthusiastic reaction. Other tender points were discovered at the nose point, which is toward the top on the middle finger, and along the lung meridian on Jack's ring finger.

THE TENDER POINTS WILL TELL

The theory behind KHT holds that hand points corresponding to ailing parts of the body will be tender when probed. By seeking out these tender points, KHT practitioners can determine the areas of the body that are suffering from pain or disease. Once these tender points are located, they become the focus of treatment.

Treatment consists of manipulating the tender points in various ways: with a probe or a similar device, with metal pellet stimulation, with gentle and focused electric stimulation, with magnets, moxibustion (the burning of herbs over the hand points), or ring therapy.

In Jack's case, Dr. Lobash manipulated or used the probe to press the nose and chest points on the middle finger, the stomach and navel points on the palm, the lung meridian on the ring finger, and the liver point on the palm of the hand. (It did hurt a little, but it was no big deal once Jack got over the shock of the first probes.) The doctor explained that he was working on the liver point because the liver is often implicated in allergies—it's not processing substances or cleansing the blood as well as it might.

After manipulating the hand points, Dr. Lobash applied metal pellet stimulation, which means that he stuck little round bandages, perhaps the size of large dimes, on the designated hand points. Each bandage held a tiny piece of metal in its center, allowing the metal to make contact with exact point on the hand that the doctor had been probing. The metals, which can be either gold, silver, or aluminum, provide constant stimulation to the hand point. Sometimes magnets are used this way, as well.

Moxibustion is a fascinating technique that's familiar to those who know about Traditional Chinese Medicine (TCM, which will be discussed in Chapter 20). A special herb, known as moxa, is placed on certain points on the body and is literally set on fire. But don't worry; it's not as dangerous as it sounds. A little pill made of the herb is attached to a cardboard-like base, which is then placed on the desired point and lit. The burning herb doesn't touch your skin. Jack's eyes widened when Dr. Lobash lit the moxa, but it just quietly burned, sending a pleasant heat right through to the hand points corresponding to Jack's chest, nose, stomach, and lungs.

Finally came the ring therapy. Acting on the theory that metals such as silver, gold, or aluminum can strengthen or dampen certain internal body activities, a ring containing the appropriate metal was placed on the finger where it would do the most good. For Jack, Dr.

Lobash slipped a silver ring on the ring finger of each hand. (The ring finger corresponds to the lung meridian.) Silver is believed to sedate the body's excess bio-energies—in Jack's case, the lungs—and therefore balance the blood flow through the radial and carotid arteries.

After all was said and done, Dr. Lobash checked Jack's pulses and found that—ta daa!—they were back in balance. The blood was flowing to his brain in the proper way, his body was well on its way to repairing itself, and theoretically, the asthmatic tightness in his chest should now begin to ease. Jack, a skeptic, was utterly surprised to find that he was, in fact, breathing more easily and felt that the asthma attack was definitely on its way out.

Two days later, while sitting in the Las Vegas airport waiting for our flight, I asked Jack what he thought about KHT now that he'd gained a little distance from the session. "Well," he told me, "I'd rather spend my time playing blackjack in one of the big casinos, but I've got to admit, I'm breathing a lot better." For him, that was a pretty strong endorsement.

FINDING A QUALIFIED PRACTITIONER

To learn more about KHT, find a practitioner, or purchase supplies, contact Dr. Dan Lobash, Ph.D., L.A., at KHT Systems, P.O. Box 5309, Hemet, California 92544; phone 877-244-4325; or check out his website, khtsystems.com.

17

Off the Tree—Healing with Herbs

Most of us think there are only two ways to get medicine, either by prescription or over-the-counter. But there is a third way, the off-the-tree approach: herbs.

An herb is any part of a plant that can be used as a medicine—the roots, stems, leaves, bark, seeds, and flowers. Up until about one hundred years ago, most medicines were made from herbs, and many of today's drugs are still herb-based. For example, the leaf of the foxglove plant is the basis of digitalis, an invaluable treatment for heart failure. Morphine is derived from opium poppies. The bark of the yew tree provides us with Taxol, a cancer drug. Aspirin is based on the same ingredients that are found in willow bark. The list goes on. And at this very moment, researchers from pharmaceutical companies all over the world are studying plants in the rain forests of South America, looking for unknown plant substances that might be able to cure our most stubborn diseases.

One of the greatest things about herbs is that they can be used in so many different ways—brewed into tea, mixed with a cream or ointment to make balm, pressed to make extract, ground into powder, or eaten whole. But whichever way you choose to take them, make no mistake: herbs *are* medicine. That's why you should only buy reputable herbal preparations off the shelf from pharmacies, grocery stores, or health food stores. Don't try to grow your own or pick herbs that you find in the wild. You need to be sure that you're getting safe, standardized doses of uncontaminated herbs.

A WORD OF WARNING

If you've got allergies, you should be very careful with herbs as they may set off an allergic reaction. Don't experiment with herbs on your own. Instead, work with a qualified herbal practitioner or a doctor, and try the preparations in the smallest possible dosage first, watching carefully for reactions. Those with asthma should be aware that the Chinese herb ma huang is the basis of ephedrine, an asthma drug, and should only be used under a doctor's supervision. Also, a few people may develop allergic reactions to the herb goldenseal or the pollen-laden flowers used to brew chamomile tea. Be careful about using either of these herbs if you're allergic to ragweed, chrysanthemums, or other members of the aster and daisy families. Also, some herbs may either interfere with medications that you're taking or interact with them, causing dangerous reactions. Be sure you tell your physician about any herbs you're either currently taking or planning to take.

HERBS FOR RESPIRATORY PROBLEMS

Asthma and certain allergies can wreak havoc on your respiratory system, causing congestion, bronchial constriction, and breathing problems. Luckily, several herbs can help loosen phlegm, improve breathing, and fight infections. But before examining those herbs, let's look at two herb terms that are specific to respiratory problems.

An *expectorant* helps you cough up troublesome mucus. There are two types of expectorants: stimulating and relaxing. Stimulating expectorants irritate the bronchial tubes, encouraging the coughing up of mucus. Relaxing expectorants calm the bronchial tubes, helping to open airways by eliminating bronchial spasms and loosening up thick plugs of mucus.

A *demulcent*, on the other hand, helps cut back on coughing. Like a cooling salve on a burn, a demulcent helps relieve irritated, sore, inflamed bronchial tissues, easing the spasms that can trigger coughing. You'll see the terms expectorant and demulcent in the descriptions of herbs that follow.

These herbs may help alleviate the respiratory symptoms associated with asthma and certain types of allergies.

Borage (*Borago officinalis*)

Way back in Roman times, borage was used to lift melancholy moods. An anti-inflammatory, it calms the respiratory system and is a good cough remedy. It also helps strengthen the immune system. Borage is usually taken as an infusion (like a tea). Make an infusion by steeping 2 teaspoons of the dried or 4 teaspoons of the fresh herb in 1 cup of boiling water for 10 to 15 minutes. Strain, add honey or sugar if desired, then drink like tea.

Elder (*Sambucus nigra*)

Also known as the European elder, common elder, or black elder, the flowers of this plant are used by herbalists to treat hay fever and other respiratory problems. Gargling with an elder flower infusion can ease a sore throat, and drinking a hot infusion made with elder flowers, yarrow, and mint can help reduce coughs, diminish symptoms of hay fever, and fight respiratory infections. (See recipe for making an infusion under Borage.)

Elecampane (*Inula helemiun*)

Also known as the wild sunflower, legend has it that this plant sprang from the tears of Helen of Troy. Formerly used to treat tuberculosis, the stimulating expectorant properties of this herb make it useful in treating asthma, bronchitis, and similar pulmonary infections. It also has powerful antibacterial and antifungal properties. An infusion of elecampane is made by mixing 1 teaspoon of the shredded root with 1 cup of cold water. Allow the tea to stand for 8 to 10 hours; then drink ⅓ cup of the infusion, heated, 3 times a day.

Eyebright (*Euphrasia officinalis*)

Just like it sounds, this herb is used to remedy sore, itchy, bloodshot eyes, but it's also an excellent treatment for problems involving the mucous membranes. Its anti-inflammatory and astringent properties make it effective as a treatment for nasal congestion, watery nasal discharge, or infection of the nasal membranes caused by hay fever and colds. Eyebright for respiratory problems is taken as an infusion. (See recipe for an infusion under Borage.)

Garlic (*Allium sativum*)

Loaded with antibiotic and antiviral properties, garlic has been used as a medicine for thousands of years, dating back at least to the time of the ancient Egyptians. Since its volatile oils are excreted mostly through the lungs, eating garlic has a positive effect on the respiratory system. It fights colds, bronchitis, the flu, and respiratory infections and helps reduce excessive production of phlegm. Many herbalists recommend eating 1 whole clove of garlic, 3 times a day, or taking garlic oil capsules.

Grindelia (*Grindelia camporum*)

An expectorant and antispasmodic, grindelia is used for hay fever, asthma, and bronchitis. This herb helps bronchial tubes relax, allowing phlegm to loosen and be expelled. Taking an infusion made from the dried herb, 3 times a day, may be recommended. (See recipe for making an infusion under Borage.)

Hyssop (*Hyssopus officinalis*)

Way back when, Hippocrates recommended hyssop for chest problems because of its expectorant qualities, and it's still used today for bronchitis, colds, and congestion. Hyssop also has antispasmodic and antiviral properties. Hyssop should be taken 3 times a day as an infusion, to ease respiratory problems. (See recipe for an making infusion under Borage.)

Licorice (*Glycyrrhiza glabra*)

Famous as a candy, licorice is both an expectorant and a demulcent. It helps you cough up mucus that may be clogging your breathing tubes, while reducing the irritation of your throat. It also contains a substance that is converted within the body into a cortisone-like material that can soothe allergic reactions. But beware, because licorice can raise blood pressure and cause your body to retain potassium and sodium. Use small doses only, and avoid licorice altogether if you are pregnant, have high blood pressure, or suffer from kidney disease. Also, don't think you'll get the medicinal effects of real licorice by eating licorice candy, because the candy contains licorice flavor only—none of the active ingredients. Licorice is taken as an infusion that is made by placing ½ to 1 teaspoon of licorice root in a cup of water. The water is brought to a boil and then allowed to simmer for 10 to 15 minutes before being strained. Drink the licorice infusion cool or warm, 3 times a day.

Lobelia (*Lobelia inflata*)

Also known as "Indian tobacco," lobelia is a popular remedy among native North Americans that contains substances that both stimulate and relax the respiratory system. Lobelia relaxes the muscles of the bronchial tubes, widening the airways, while encouraging expulsion of mucus. This herb is taken as an infusion, using ¼ to ½ teaspoon of dried leaves per cup of boiling water.

Marshmallow (*Althea officinalis*)

Marshmallow is both a demulcent, with wonderful soothing and healing properties, and a mild expectorant. The leaf is used for respiratory problems, as it eases bronchitis; irritating coughs; infections of the mucous membranes; and inflamed tissues in the chest, throat, and sinuses. The infusion is generally taken 3 times a day. (See recipe for making an infusion under Borage.)

Mullein (*Verbascum thapus*)

Mullein has a reputation for being one of the best normalizers of the entire chest area. It tones the mucous membranes, reduces inflammation, and encourages production and expulsion of mucus, making it useful in the treatment of asthma and other respiratory problems. Mullein is generally taken as an infusion three times a day. (See recipe for making an infusion under Borage.)

Pill-Bearing Spurge (*Euphorbiaceae*)

One of its alternate names, asthma weed, tells it all. This tropical herb helps ease asthma, bronchitis, and hay fever symptoms by relaxing the smooth muscles in the bronchial tubes, clearing mucus from the respiratory tract, and fighting bronchial infections. An infusion of ½ to

1 teaspoon of dried leaves steeped in 1 cup boiling water for 10 to 15 minutes, taken 3 times a day, is usually recommended.

Skunk Cabbage (*Symplocarpus foetidus*)

Used for asthma, bronchitis, and whooping cough, this smelly herb is also effective at soothing an overstressed nervous system. An antispasmodic and expectorant, skunk cabbage can help ease chest tightness and irritating coughs. An infusion is made from the root of this herb, using ½ to 1 teaspoon of root per cup of water. Beware of fresh skunk cabbage, however, as it can cause blistering.

Thyme (*Thymus vulgaris*)

Thyme leaves can benefit the respiratory system in many ways with its antimicrobial, antispasmodic, and expectorant qualities. Drinking an infusion made from thyme leaves is believed to be helpful in treating bronchitis, whooping cough, and asthma. (See recipe for making an infusion under Borage.)

White Horehound (*Marrubium vulgare*)

Long a treatment for digestive and liver ailments, fever, and malaria, an infusion made from the leaves and flowers of this stimulating expectorant is prized for its ability to relax the smooth muscles of the bronchioles and promote both the production and expulsion of mucus. An infusion, made from ½ to 1 teaspoon of the dried herb per cup of boiling water, is usually taken 3 times a day.

Wild Cherry Bark (*Prunus serotina*)

Used for irritating, continuous, or nervous coughing, this herb helps relax the coughing reflex. It's used for bronchitis, whooping cough, and asthma. The infusion is made of 1 teaspoon dried bark, steeped in 1 cup of boiling water for 10 to 15 minutes, and is generally taken 3 times a day.

HERBS FOR ALLERGIES

Although you'll want to be careful not to exacerbate your condition, there are a few herbs that may ease your symptoms and help your body start to quiet down.

Chamomile (*Matricaria chamomilla*)

A cool infusion, taken as a drink or used as a cool compress, may help relieve the itchiness of hives. (See recipe for making an infusion under Borage.) Avoid chamomile if you're allergic to ragweed, chrysanthemums, or other members of the aster and daisy families.

Chickweed (*Stellaria media*)

This herb can have a soothing effect on eczema, hives, or other itching caused by allergic reactions. It is usually used externally, often combined with marshmallow, in ointment form. It can also be used as a poultice, and a strong infusion can be added to the bathwater to ease itching. Or chickweed can be taken internally as an infusion, primarily to relieve rheumatism. (See recipe for making an infusion under Borage, but only steep for 5 minutes.)

Marigold (*Calendula officianalis*)

Helpful in soothing eczema and other skin irritations, an infusion is made by combining 1 ounce of marigold petals with 2 cups of boiling water. Steep for 5 minutes then strain. It's generally recommended that you drink this concoction 3 times a day. Marigold is also available as a topical treatment in the form of calendula cream.

Marshmallow (*Althea officinalis*)

Both the leaf and the root of this herb are very soothing to internal and external tissues. Poultices can be made from the chopped herb, compresses from the infusion, or the infusion can be taken internally. (See recipe for making an infusion under Borage.)

Meadowsweet (*Filipendula ulmaria*)

This herb contains aspirin-like compounds that ease inflammation, reduce fever, and quell pain. It's particularly helpful as a digestive remedy, soothing membranes of the digestive tract, and easing nausea. Meadowsweet flowers and leaves are made into an infusion, which is generally recommended 3 times a day or as needed. (See recipe for making an infusion under Borage.)

Nettles (*Urtica dioica*)

An infusion made from nettles may quell some allergic reactions and is useful in treating childhood eczema. The infusion is prepared by using 1 to 3 teaspoons of the dried herb per cup of boiling water, steeping for 10 to 15 minutes. Drink 3 times per day.

HERBS TO EASE TENSION

Tension, stress, and anxiety can make asthma and allergies even worse. But once you're in the throes of an asthma attack or allergic reaction, it's hard to remain calm. These herbs may help you relax, center yourself, and keep your emotions from spiraling out of control.

Chamomile (*Matricaria chamomilla*)

Probably the most popular and widely known herbal remedy, an infusion made from chamomile flowers acts as a gentle sedative that also eases inflammation. Used extensively for anxiety and insomnia, chamomile can also soothe sore throats when used as a gargle and speed recovery of mucous membrane infections when used with a steam inhaler. For anxiety, an infusion made from 2 teaspoons of the dried flowers per 1 cup of boiling water steeped for 5 to 10 minutes is often suggested. For steam inhalation, put ½ cup of the dried flowers into 2 liters of boiling water. When the water has cooled sufficiently, put a towel over your head (and the pot) and inhale the steam for 5 minutes. Be careful not to burn yourself when inhaling the steam. Avoid chamomile if you're allergic to ragweed, chrysanthemums, or other members of the aster and daisy families.

Hops (*Lumulus lupulus*)

This herb, long treasured for its role in making beer, is also known for its ability to sedate and aid in relaxation when taken as a tea. It's used to treat insomnia, tension, anxiety, and restlessness. An infusion is made from 1 teaspoon of dried flowers steeped in 1 cup of boiling water for 10 to 15 minutes is often recommended at night to induce sleep—or any time tension and anxiety are problematic.

Scullcap (*Scutellaria laterifolia*)

Anxiety, depression, and insomnia, all common side effects of allergies, can be eased by scullcap, which acts as a nerve tonic and sedative. It's also an antispasmodic, making it helpful in the treatment of asthma. An infusion, taken 3 times a day, is recommended to ease tension and aid in relaxing the bronchial tubes. (See recipe for making an infusion under Borage.) But beware. Large doses can trigger irregular heartbeat, dizziness, and other problems.

Valerian (*Valeriana officinalis*)

The root of this herb smells a little bit like stinky gym socks, but it's one of the most useful herbs available for reducing tension, easing anxiety, promoting safe and healing sleep, and relaxing muscle spasms. An infusion is made by pouring 1 cup of boiling water over 1 to 2 teaspoons of the ground root for 10 to 15 minutes. Valerian can also be taken in capsule form if you can't abide the smelly tea.

Wild Lettuce (*Lactuca virosa*)

A cousin to the kind of lettuce that we put in salads, wild lettuce contains a milky substance that looks like opium and is used in soaps, shampoos, and teas. This substance can help alleviate anxiety and fear, two major side effects of asthma and allergies that can increase the duration and intensity of your reaction. But beware; too much wild lettuce is poisonous. It's generally recommended that one take an infusion made from 1 to 2 teaspoons of dried leaves steeped in 1 cup of boiling water for 10 to 15 minutes, 3 times a day.

FINDING A QUALIFIED HERBAL PRACTITIONER

Don't try to go it alone when experimenting with herbs and herbal preparations. Instead, work with a qualified herbal expert. To get a list of naturopathic physicians qualified in herbal medicine, contact the American Association of Naturopathic Physicians at 602 Valley Street, Suite 105, Seattle, Washington 98109; phone 206-298-0126; or visit their wesite, naturopathic.org.

18

Embrace the Enemy with Homeopathy

The literal translation of homeopathy is "similar suffering," because the basic principle of homeopathy involves treating a disease with tiny amounts of the very same thing that causes the disease. This approach isn't as crazy as it sounds. Your medical doctor has probably already treated your allergies in a homeopathic way. Allergy shots slowly help you build up a tolerance to certain allergens by introducing a little bit of the offending substance over and over again. Eventually, if all goes well, you no longer develop allergic symptoms when exposed to moderate amounts of that substance.

Homeopathy dates back to the late 1700s, when Dr. Samuel Hahnemann decided that standard Western medicine was way too risky and not nearly effective enough, mainly because of the powerful drugs that were used to suppress symptoms. They just masked the effects of the problem, rather than attacking the problem at its root. Not only that, the drugs had too many side effects, some of which were worse than the disease itself. Eventually, Dr. Hahnemann stumbled upon, tested, and refined a new approach that was based upon the idea that "like cures like." Instead of using opposites, powerful drugs to stamp out symptoms, he gave his patients a little bit more of the thing that caused the disease as a way of stimulating the body to cure itself.

The theory behind homeopathy is similar to that of the modern vaccine, which introduces a dead or weakened version of certain germs. The immune system then forms antibodies to these invaders so that when the real germs invade, the body is all ready to launch an attack. This method has made it possible to practically wipe out certain diseases, like smallpox and rubella.

Something similar happens with homeopathy, although you aren't given a version of the germ until *after* you become ill. Once you develop symptoms, the homeopathic physician will give you very small doses of substances that cause similar symptoms in healthy people. This will encourage your body to rally its defenses and defeat the disease. Thus, like will cure like.

To illustrate, suppose you're in the midst of an allergic reaction to pollen. Your eyes are watering up a storm, your nose is running faster than an Olympic sprinter, and your head feels like Muhammad Ali is pummeling away from the inside. Your homeopath will treat you with very small doses of substances called *remedies* that actually cause watery eyes, runny noses, and headaches in healthy people. But not any old homeopathic remedy for allergy symptoms will do the trick; the remedy must be closely matched to your body's unique makeup.

According to homeopathic theory, the allergy symptoms that drive you crazy are not the real problem; they're just outward manifestations of the deeper physical, mental, or emotional problems within. Somehow your basic constitutional makeup, your very essence, has been disturbed. The solution lies in mapping out your essence, then using the homeopathic remedies that most closely match your essence to help it return to normal.

To figure out your essence and prescribe a constitutional remedy, the homeopathic physician will need to do an in-depth interview with you. He or she will ask you questions about your eating habits, how well you sleep, about your home life, your family, your emotional life, and your work; about the stressors in your life, whether you're a cold weather or hot weather person, and so on. You'll also be asked about your symptoms; what you were doing when they struck; where you were; what you were eating; if the problem seems to be worse in the morning, afternoon, evening, or night; if it occurs more often at work than at home; if it happens when you're upset; and so on.

Armed with this information (and a lot more), the homeopath will zero in on the physical, mental, or emotional problems that are plaguing you. Then you will be given the remedy that's most closely attuned to your essence, one that strikes at the root of your problem. You may also be given other remedies to help with your allergy or asthma symptoms, but these aren't considered essential remedies. They're just supposed to help you get through the day or sleep through the night.

There are about two thousand remedies made from tiny amounts of animal, plant, or mineral substances, all of which are highly diluted. Homeopaths believe that the more diluted the remedy, the stronger it is, and that shaking them vigorously will make them more effective. Homeopathic remedies come in pill, powder, tablet, liquid, or granule form.

One popular homeopathic remedy for respiratory allergies, allium cepa (commonly known as red onion), is a good example of the basic homeopathic principle: in healthy people, the onion causes the eyes to water and the nose to run, but does just the opposite in those who already have these problems. But not everyone with allergy-driven nose and eye problems will benefit from allium cepa because it has to be suited to the problem. Allium cepa works best if the eyes are already red and tearing, the nasal discharge is burning, the discharge increases in a warm room and decreases in fresh air, the nose is raw and tingly, and sneezing is violent.

In contrast, for burning tears, reddened eyes, and a nonburning nasal discharge that worsens in the wind or when lying down, the recommended remedy is euphrasia, which comes from the herb eyebright. As you can see, homeopathy can be a bit complex. With that in mind, glance through the following remedies, but rely on a trained homeopath to tell you what's right for you.

Homeopathic Remedies for Allergic Skin Rashes

- **Anacardium (Anacardium)**—for rashes (usually on the face) with large blisters filled with yellow fluid
- **Ars alb (Arsenicum album)**—for skin rashes that burn and are accompanied by restlessness
- **Bovista (Bovista)**—for skin rashes that spring up overnight, often following excitement, and are accompanied by diarrhea
- **Bryonia (Bryonia alba)**—for dry, fine, bumpy rashes on the chest, upper back, or face accompanied by thirst for large amounts of cold water
- **Calc carb (Cacarea carbonica-ostrearum)**—for chronic rashes that get worse when you drink milk
- **Croton tig (Croton tigium)**—for acute inflammation, itching, and blistering, usually affecting the genitals, eyes, or scalp
- **Dulcamara (Dulcamara)**—for chronic rashes that get worse as fall gives way to winter
- **Nat mur (Natrum muriaticum)**—for rashes that itch more when you exercise or otherwise exert yourself
- **Rhus tox (Rhus toxicodendron)**—for poison ivy, poison oak, poison sumac, or other rashes that itch, burn, and are aggravated by scratching, open air, nighttime, or the warmth of the bed
- **Sepia (Sepia)**—for dry rashes or rashes with very tiny blisters, eased by being in a warm room but aggravated by a warm bed

Homeopathic Remedies for Hay Fever

- **Allium cepa (Allium cepa)**—when the problem is worse in the evening and indoors, and there is a headache and frequent sneezing
- **Arundo (Arundo mauritanica)**—for itchy eyes, nose, and soft palate.

- **Dulcamara (Dulcamara)**—when hay fever strikes in the late summer or fall, the eyes swell and tear, resting indoors helps, and rain makes everything worse
- **Euphrasia (Euphrasia)**—for red, inflamed, watery, or infected eyes and a nonirritating nasal discharge
- **Gelsemium (Gelsemium)**—when symptoms are worse in the morning, the eyes feel hot and look bloodshot, there is a burning nasal discharge, the face feels hot, and the limbs ache
- **Pulsatilla (Pulsatilla)**—for stuffed ears and infected eyes
- **Sabadilla (Sabadilla)**—for typical hay fever symptoms such as itchy, watery eyes, runny nose, and sneezing
- **Sanguinaria (Sanguinaria)**—for dry, burning eyes, unquenchable thirst, and a nose that is alternately dry and runny.

Homeopathic Remedies for Asthma

- **Aconite (Aconitum napellus)**—for attacks that spring up suddenly following cold, dry winds
- **Ant tart (Antimonium tartaricum)**—when the bronchial tubes are filled with mucus and one is very short of breath, weak, and drowsy
- **Caladium (Caladium)**—when the asthma strikes in conjunction with, or alternates with, a skin rash
- **Cuprum met (Cuprum metallicum)**—when there is a suffocating feeling in the middle of the night and excessive coughing turns the face blue
- **Hypericum (Hypericum)**—when a change in the weather can trigger an attack
- **Ipecac (Ipecacuanha)**—for a dry, spasmodic, unproductive cough with wheezing and a shortage of breath during exertion
- **Nat sulph (Natrum sulphuricum)**—for shortness of breath, rattling in the chest, or for asthma associated with humidity

- **Urtica (Urtica urens)**—a general anti-allergenic that reduces mucus production.

Traditional homeopaths will give you just one remedy at a time, then wait to see if it works. If not, they'll try another. Other, more modern homeopaths may give several remedies at once.

Remedies must be taken with a clean mouth—that is, don't eat or drink anything or use toothpaste for at least ten minutes before you take the remedy. Powdered remedies should be sprinkled right on the tongue; pills should be chewed or put underneath the tongue and allowed to dissolve.

Although there aren't stacks of scientific evidence that support the effectiveness of homeopathy, millions of people—including members of the British royal family—use it regularly and are satisfied with the results. You may not see instantaneous improvement when you take homeopathic remedies because it can take awhile for the medicine to help you overcome the constitutional upset. And, in some cases, the symptoms can actually grow worse at first, as your body begins to battle the problem.

FINDING A QUALIFIED HOMEOPATH

Homeopathic remedies have become so popular that they're currently available in many major supermarkets and drug stores. But don't self-administer them for serious ailments like allergies or asthma. Using homeopathy to balance the body and the emotions at a deep cellular level is a complex process. You'll need to see a trained homeopathic physician to find out which remedy or combination of remedies is right for you. You can find one by contacting the National Center for Homeopathy at 801 N. Fairfax Street, Suite 306, Alexandria, Virginia 22314; phone 703-548-7790; or visit their website, homeo pathic.org.

19 Ayurvedic Medicine

Is your hay fever driving you crazy? Odds are you've got too much air. Is asthma making it difficult for you to breathe? You've probably got too much water—or so say practitioners of Ayurvedic medicine. Those who endorse the ancient healing system known as Ayurveda believe that the human body, like the universe, is composed of a mixture of elements: earth, water, fire, air, and ether. In the body, these five essential components combine in different ways to create the three primary life forces (*doshas*), called *vata*, *pitta*, and *kapha*.

Born of a mixture of air and ether, vata is charged with the primary responsibility for respiration, circulation, elimination, the nervous system, muscles, and movements within the body's fluid and cells.

Springing from fire and earth, pitta oversees digestion, chemical reactions inside the body's fluids and cells, and other metabolic reactions. Skin color, temperature, intelligence, and understanding are all under pitta's sway.

A combination of water and ether, kapha takes responsibility for growth, as well as the protection of the body from invaders that can enter via the mouth, nose, and so forth. Kapha also protects through its influence on the body fluids that cushion the brain, keep the skin moist, and ensure that the joints are well lubricated.

Depending on how earth, water, fire, air, and ether have combined in your body, you're either a vata, pitta, or kapha type. But it's not as simple as saying that you belong strictly to one of three categories and that's that. Most people tend to be one type or another, but many are a cross between two or even three types. And figuring out your doshic makeup can be difficult: there isn't a simple blood test or check-off exam you can take. Instead, an Ayurvedic physician must make that determination by asking you a lot of questions about your habits and lifestyle, examining you from head to toe, and factoring in the influences of the seven body tissues (*dhatus*), three types of wastes (*malas*), and the energy of metabolism. It's quite a complex equation. And it doesn't take much to upset the doshic balance—poor diet, stress, lack of exercise, or spiritual troubles can all disturb your very essence and pave the way to illness.

AYURVEDIC VERSUS WESTERN MEDICINE

Born thousands of years ago in India, Ayurvedic healing is a horse of a different color. It may be easiest to understand by comparing it to Western medicine, the kind we're most familiar with in North America. For example:

- Western medicine is based on the idea that germs or genetic problems cause disease; Ayurveda looks to the essential imbalance in the body's elemental constitution and energy flow, as well as the psychological and spiritual causes of physical distress.
- Western medicine typically attacks disease by literally destroying it with strong drugs; Ayurveda looks past the symptoms in an attempt to understand the essential weakness that allowed disease to flourish in the first place.
- Western medicine sees each patient as being pretty much the same, except for age, sex, weight, and genetic makeup; Ayurveda differentiates us according to life force.

- Western medicine believes that outside interference is necessary to cure disease; Ayurveda argues that the body is its own best doctor.
- Western medicine focuses almost exclusively on drugs and surgery; Ayurveda employs a variety of means to help the body heal itself, including diet, herbs, yoga, massage, prayer, meditation, and color therapy.

CURING THE ALLERGIC IMBALANCE

We don't have enough space to explore the Ayurvedic treatments for every kind of allergy, so let's look at hay fever as an example of the way Ayurvedic physicians approach treatment. This allergy usually strikes vata-type people, who will often suffer from headaches, unproductive coughs, insomnia, and anxiety. If the hay fever is of the pitta type, it will produce rashes; burning, red eyes; fever; thirst; a yellowish nasal discharge; and blood toxicity, while those with the kapha type will feel heavy and dull and will discharge either white or clear phlegm.

The goal is to restore the doshic balance, allowing the body to heal itself. Treatment may begin with a detoxifying diet designed to rid the body of impurities, strengthen the immune system, and regulate the body's heat. Foods that encourage the production of mucus, such as milk, must be avoided.

To help restore respiratory system strength and clear the sinuses, a variety of herbs may be prescribed: ashwagandha, astragalus, bala, bayberry, cloves, ginseng, ginger, gotu kola, peppermint, sage, and wintergreen. Basil tea is helpful for everyone, while cilantro and coriander may be especially helpful for pitta-type hay fever. For kapha types, dry ginger powder may be recommended as snuff.

In addition to diet and herbs, the Ayurvedic doctor may prescribe changes in lifestyle habits, such as exercise, meditation, enemas, herbs, purging, sweating, breathing techniques, gem therapy, or chanting.

If all goes according to plan, the individualized program will restore the doshic balance and the body will heal itself.

Gem therapy is a fascinating part of Ayurveda, and is based on the idea that different colors affect the body in different ways. The ruby, for example, strengthens the heart, increases energy, and revives the body's internal fire. It increases pitta while decreasing kapha and vata, so it can help restore doshic balance. Emeralds have different effects, harmonizing vata, slightly increasing kapha, and decreasing pitta. Emeralds also restore the nervous system to health, increase energy, and strengthen the lungs.

While gems may be interesting, another part of Ayurveda—chanting—can be fun. Chanting is often combined with yoga, using different chants for different purposes. You assume a particular yoga posture, take a deep breath, and slowly exhale while vocalizing a prescribed sound (a mantra). You continue making one long sound until you run out of breath. "Om," for example, is an all-purpose chant that cleanses the mind while energizing and opening up the body. "Ram" promotes strength and peace, and helps relieve problems associated with excess vata. "Hreem" speeds detoxification, and a wide array of other mantras also have their strengths and applications.

FINDING A QUALIFIED AYURVEDIC PRACTITIONER

Reading a book on Ayurvedic medicine is a great way to acquaint yourself with this healing art, but eventually you'll need to work with a skilled Ayurvedic doctor. For more information and a list of referrals, contact the National Institute of Ayurvedic Medicine at 584 Miltown Road, Brewster, New York 10509; phone 888-246-6426; or visit their website, niam.com.

20

Traditional Chinese Medicine

Dark and light, cold and hot, giving and receiving, exertion and rest. The dance of the contradictory and the balance between perpetual opposites keep us healthy, according to Traditional Chinese Medicine (TCM), an ancient healing art.

The opposing camps of the universe are *yin* and *yang*. Yin, the female principle, is dark and cold, while yang, the male principle, is light and hot. Yin and yang are everywhere and in everything; in a sense, they are everything, since everything is composed of a balanced measure of these two forces. But if that balance should become upset, the flow of internal chi (energy) will also be disturbed and we will become ill.

But balancing the yin and yang is only part of the equation. Chinese medicine groups the body's organs into five elements not found in Western medicine, and these elements must also be balanced:

1. Fire, related to the heart (which is a yin organ) and the small intestine (which is a yang organ)
2. Earth, related to the spleen (yin) and stomach (yang)
3. Metal, related to the lungs (yin) and large intestine (yang)

4. Water, related to the kidney (yin) and bladder (yang)
5. Wood, related to the liver (yin) and gallbladder (yang)

YOUR VISIT TO A DOCTOR OF CHINESE MEDICINE

As in Ayurvedic medicine, practitioners of Chinese medicine have some ways of viewing disease and its diagnosis that will seem unusual to those of us used to Western medicine. The doctor will ask you numerous questions about your symptoms, appetite, bowel habits, emotions, and more. He will study your skin, tongue, eyes, fingernails, and other body parts very carefully and inspect your stool and urine. The sounds made by your breathing and bowels, as well as your voice, will give clues. So will your pulse, which retains much greater importance in TCM than in Western medicine.

The eventual diagnosis may be something like "a disturbance in the flow of energy caused by too much phlegm." Phlegm here does not mean mucus. Instead, phlegm is the disharmony, the imbalance that is disrupting your body and emotions. This may be due to a weakness of the lungs, spleen, or kidneys; poor diet; or other factors. The many questions the doctor asks will help pinpoint the cause of the problem.

Once the source of your problem has been diagnosed, the doctor will use a variety of means to restore balance within your body, including nutrition, acupuncture, ear acupuncture, herbs, spices, and massage. The treatment may seem a little odd to you at first, but remember that the goal is to restore harmony rather than suppress symptoms.

SOME TCM TREATMENTS FOR ALLERGIES

Traditional Chinese medicine has several ways of treating allergies, including the following.

Acupuncture

Often the spearhead of treatment (so to speak) in TCM, very fine needles are inserted into various points on your body, including your back, arms, wrists, and hands. The doctor of Chinese medicine tries to restore harmony and the flow of energy within your body by placing these needles along special meridians (body channels through which energy flows) that influence the problem organs or areas. If your allergy manifests in the skin, for example, acupuncture may be performed on points that correspond to the meridians that have an affect on the skin, such as the lung and colon meridians. Specific points on the lower arms, wrists, and hands may also be targeted. For allergies that show up as stuffy noses or breathing problems, points on the face, hands, upper chest, upper back, and base of the neck are often used.

Ear Acupuncture

The doctor may also perform ear acupuncture, which is based on the idea that manipulating specific points on the ears will trigger beneficial reactions in the body. The ear is believed to contain a map of the body, with the head in the earlobe, many internal organs by the opening of the ear, and the fingers and toes at the top.

Acupressure

The theories of acupuncture also govern acupressure, but instead of needles, the doctor will use his or her fingers, thumbs, hands, elbows, and even feet to stimulate the proper acupuncture points on your body. (See the explanation of shiatsu, which is another name for acupressure, in Chapter 15.)

Diet

In addition to acupuncture, ear acupuncture, or acupressure, your treatment will most likely include diet, which is an important component of this ancient healing art. But this won't be our kind of diet, broken down according to calories, fat, carbohydrates, protein, and so forth. In Chinese medicine, foods are included in various dietary therapies because of their flavors, energies, and organic actions. Your doctor will devise a diet for you that promotes balance from within, and he or she may also suggest foods that are especially helpful for easing allergy symptoms, like cork silk, hawthorn fruit, pumpkin, and tangerine. These foods help reduce the nasal inflammation, runny nose, and chest congestion seen with some allergies, as well as the symptoms of allergic asthma.

Herbs and Spices

Herbs and spices will play an important role in your treatment. From more than three thousand Chinese medicine herbal products, your doctor may choose herbs like ginseng, which is a good general tonic; ginger, to help cleanse and purify your body; Chinese gentian or peony root for eczema; and Chinese angelica, for anxiety and associated symptoms.

FINDING A QUALIFIED TCM PRACTITIONER

Chinese medicine is nothing to fool with. Acupuncture is an invasive therapy and Chinese herbs can be very strong and may have side effects. That's why it's important to avoid diagnosing or treating yourself and to make sure you work with a qualified doctor of Oriental medicine. To find one, contact the National Certification Commission for Acupuncture and Oriental Medicine (NCCAOM) at 11 Canal Center Plaza, Suite 330, Alexandria, Virginia 22314; phone 703-548-9004; or visit their website, nccaom.org.

21
Aromatherapy

You might think that taking a big whiff of some aromatic substance is just about the worst thing you can do to your hyperactive respiratory system. For some people this may be true, but many have found that inhaling certain natural fragrances and other aromas can actually bring about an inner calm that does much to promote the healing of their asthma or allergies.

Long before mankind had access to "nighttime sniffling, sneezing, and runny nose" medicines, aromas were used to treat a variety of ailments. Way back in 2690 B.C., the use of various aromas to cure diseases was written about in the *Chinese Yellow Emperor Book of Internal Medicine*. The ancient Egyptians treated asthma and other problems with a fragrance called *kyphi*, a blend of cinnamon, cypress, myrrh, frankincense, and other herbs. The aromas of various herbs were also used as medicines during the Greek and Roman eras, the Middle Ages, and the Industrial Era—in fact, right up until the early part of the twentieth century, when drugs became the superstars of medical protocol. Even then, if your mother was like mine, she probably treated your colds by making you inhale the aroma of menthol from a vaporizer or from a thick, gooey chest ointment.

THE SECRET IS IN THE OILS

In recent years, the healing art of aromatherapy, as it's now known, has become wildly popular. It's based on the inhalation of the fragrances produced by various essential oils. These oils are made from the very concentrated extracts of herbs, flowers, grasses, shrubs, and trees and are designed to balance, relax, and revitalize the body, spirit, and mind. You can enjoy the benefits of the essential oils by inhaling their fragrances, applying the oils to your body via massage, adding them to your bathwater, or, in some cases, even ingesting them in the form of tea. But using just any old fragrant oil won't do. The oils must come from specific plants and be taken from the plants via one of three processes: steam distillation, peel pressure, or solvent extraction. The essential oils that result are very concentrated, aromatic, and full of various organic compounds that affect the human mind, body, or spirit. (There's a competing discipline called aromacology that believes that manufactured artificial aromas are just as effective, but die-hard aromatherapy fans beg to differ.)

Essential oils have certain undisputed effects on the body. Some have antimicrobial, antifungal, or antiseptic abilities; others have congestion-clearing or wound-healing properties that function as anti-inflammatories. Certain oils can also help increase circulation or raise or lower the blood pressure. Some of the best-known results brought about by essential oils have to do with psychological states of mind—they can produce a sense of calmness, sedation, euphoria, or excitement.

Only the highest-quality essential oils should be used for aromatherapy, as many of the lesser quality oils are adulterated with chemicals or synthetic additives. Make sure you purchase your oils from a reputable source (e.g., an accredited aromatherapist). You may find it expensive, especially if you're interested in using several oils, but because you'll only use a couple of drops at a time, a bottle should last for quite awhile.

It's easy to use essential oils. Bring a pot of water to a boil; cool it slightly, then add a few drops of the oil to the water. When the steam has cooled at bit, put a towel over your head and the pot and inhale the aroma as it rises with the steam. The oils can be added to your bath or a put into a humidifier to distribute the aroma throughout an entire room. The same effect can be achieved with an aromatic diffuser. If that sounds like too much trouble, one of the simplest ways of inhaling aromas is to buy a natural products aroma inhaler. It looks something like a tube of lipstick; you pull off the cover and inhale the aroma that wafts out of the inner cylinder. No preparation is necessary.

My favorite way of receiving aromatherapy is via massage. Essential oils are never applied directly to the skin (they are too irritating) but are mixed into a larger amount of a carrier oil such as soybean or sesame oil. Then, this combination of oils is applied to the therapist's palms and transferred to your skin during massage. You lie on the massage table as the tension is kneaded out of your muscles, and you simultaneously inhale the relaxing, sedating aroma of, say, lavender.

AROMAS FOR ALLERGIES AND ASTHMA

The following essential oils are sometimes used to ease allergies and asthma.

Benzoin

This oil smells a little like vanilla and comes from the resin of the benzoin tree, which is native to Java, Sumatra, and Thailand. Benzoin essential oil has antiseptic and expectorant properties and can help ease asthma, bronchitis, coughs, skin irritations, and wounds.

Bergamot

Taken from the rind of a citrus fruit that looks like a pear-shaped orange, this sweet, citrusy, floral-scented essential oil has antiseptic and expectorant properties that can help ease respiratory tract infections, speed wound healing, clear up psoriasis, and help strengthen the body overall.

Cypress

Taken from tall, cone-shaped trees of Eastern origin that now grow in the Mediterranean area or in English parks, cypress has a woody, slightly spicy aroma that has antiseptic, antispasmodic properties, making it helpful in treating asthma, spasmodic cough, whooping cough, and a runny nose.

Eucalyptus

These supertall trees, which are native to Australia, have long, sword-shaped leaves that contain an aromatic oil that smells something like camphor. Eucalyptus oil has antiseptic, antispasmodic, and expectorant properties, making it useful in the battle against asthma, bronchitis, catarrh, colds, cough, sinusitis, and throat infections.

Hyssop

This herb, found in hilly, warm, arid places, has been used for centuries and is even mentioned in the Bible. The light yellowish oil that's taken from its thin, pointy leaves is found in costly perfumes and liqueurs and smells something like a combination of thyme and geranium. It has antiseptic, antispasmodic, expectorant, and tonic properties that can help fight asthma, bronchitis, catarrh, cough, dermatitis, eczema, whooping cough, and other problems.

Lavender

The oil taken from this plant's flowers was used by ancient Romans in their baths, which may explain why its name comes from the Latin word for "wash." Today, this fragrant oil is used in many colognes, soaps, potpourris, sachets, and air fresheners. The essential oil has antidepressant, antispasmodic, and sedative properties and is used for asthma, bites, bronchitis, dermatitis, eczema, influenza, laryngitis, psoriasis, throat infections, whooping cough, and immune system deficiency.

Marjoram

The savory leaves of this herb were favored by the ancient Greeks and used as medicines and perfumes. They named it margaron, which means "pearl." Marjoram essential oil produces a warming, relaxing aroma, with antiseptic, antispasmodic, expectorant, and sedative properties. Today it's used for asthma, colds, headaches, nervous tension, and other ailments.

Patchouli

This herb, native to India, produces a deep reddish-brown oil that's thick enough to use as glue and smells a bit like an old musty attic. It has antidepressant, antiseptic, and sedative qualities and may aid in the treatment of allergies and inflammation.

Peppermint

This fragrant and familiar herb is used to flavor toothpaste, mouthwash, antacids, desserts, and many other items that we use on a daily basis. Its essential oil has antiseptic, antispasmodic, expectorant, and nervine properties, making it useful in treating asthma, bronchitis, colds, cough, dermatitis, toothaches, sinus congestion, and other problems.

Rosemary

Burned as incense by the ancients or used as a way to fumigate sick rooms, rosemary has been employed as an herbal medicine for centuries to improve the memory, strengthen the nerves, and warm the heart. Its warm, piney, camphor-like scent is invigorating and has antiseptic, antispasmodic, and stimulating qualities. Asthma, bronchitis, colds, and whooping cough may all benefit from the use of this essential oil.

BEFORE YOU TRY AROMATHERAPY . . .

Some essential oils can cause allergic reactions. If you like the idea of trying aromatherapy for your asthma or respiratory allergies, do so only under the guidance of your doctor. Then, begin experimenting with aromas with a trained aromatherapist, at least at first, until you know how your body will react to the different aromas. Be sure to tell him in advance about your conditions. Also, don't use aromatherapy (in any form) while you're having an asthma attack. You may develop a reaction to the oil and find it even harder to breathe.

FINDING A QUALIFIED AROMATHERAPIST

To find a certified aromatherapist, contact the National Association for Holistic Aromatherapy (NAHA), P.O. Box 17622, Boulder, Colorado 80308; phone 303-258-3791; or visit their website, naha.org.

22

Talk It Out with Psychotherapy

There seems to be little doubt that the mind exerts a powerful effect upon the body—sometimes for the better, sometimes for the worse. Although we used to believe that the physical and the mental/emotional were completely separate entities, it's becoming more and more obvious that the two are inseparable. The brain is linked to the immune system and the endocrine system by a complex electrochemical system, sending and receiving millions of messages that rocket through your body in the blink of an eye. These messages can instantly alter the secretion of hormones, neuropeptides, immune system "soldiers," and other substances made by the glands. This, in turn, affects your moods, resistance to disease, mental sharpness, fatigue levels, and the amount of pain you feel, among other things. What does this mean to you? It means that what you think and how you feel emotionally can make a big difference to your physical health. So it's not surprising that feeling frustrated or discouraged by the onset of yet another asthma attack can make the problem even worse, or that an allergic rash may become more intense and long-lasting when you're upset.

THE "TALKING THERAPY"

Just the fact that you have asthma or allergies can be such a stressor in your life that it automatically lowers your resistance and makes your condition worse. It's easy to get caught in this vicious circle: your allergy stresses you out, and that makes you develop more intense symptoms, which makes you even more stressed out. How can you break the chain? The answer may lie in psychotherapy, the "talking therapy." Talking your problems through with a person who has been trained to listen, help you understand your behavior, and guide you toward positive solutions might make an enormous difference in both your mental and physical health. Don't get me wrong—I'm not trying to tell you that your asthma or allergies are all in your mind or the result of some sort of mental imbalance. But, because stress and emotional upsets do play a major part in asthma and allergies, talking to someone about the problems and challenges can and does help many people. If nothing else, it can be a way for you to unburden yourself and release some stress.

KINDS OF PSYCHOTHERAPY

There are lots of different kinds of psychotherapy, but the most important thing will be the relationship that you develop with your therapist. You'll need to feel completely comfortable with this person so that you'll be able to relax and reveal your innermost thoughts. Respect for the therapist's knowledge, wisdom, and attitudes will also play a big part in the relationship. And you'll really need to "click" with the therapist on a personal level. In short, not just anybody is going to be a good match for you, and you may need to try out several therapists before you find the one who seems right. If you just don't feel right about the psychotherapist, or you feel you're not getting anywhere after several sessions, try someone else. The right person is out there somewhere, if you're patient and persistent enough to find her.

That said, I've listed some of the main kinds of psychotherapy, just to give you an idea of what's available.

Behavioral Therapy

Based on the theory that all behavior is learned, which means it can also be "un-learned," this form of psychotherapy uses *operant conditioning* (rewarding desirable behavior while ignoring undesirable behavior) and a gradual exposure, in a controlled environment, to the things that are unduly feared. The fear of flying is often treated this way. At first, you imagine yourself getting into an airplane; later you actually board, sit down, and fasten your seatbelt. Eventually, you get into a flight simulator. One day you might actually take a real flight.

Cognitive Behavioral Therapy

This therapy focuses on the way you look at the world, which is believed to affect your emotions and, as a result, the way you behave. If you have a negative view of yourself, you may begin to form irrational beliefs about yourself and your relationships with others. The therapist tries to alter these faulty perceptions and thoughts about yourself and the world around you, to teach you to see things more positively and rationally. The techniques used include reality testing, thought substitution, role-playing, and teaching new coping strategies.

Psychoanalysis

This therapy, made famous by Sigmund Freud, is based on the idea that all anxiety and unhappiness stem from the subconscious mind. Early emotional experiences may be so deeply buried (repressed) that you can't remember them, but they will surface at some point as anxiety, depression, migraine headaches, or stress-related conditions like asthma or allergies. The psychoanalyst may ask you to lie on the proverbial couch and just say whatever comes to mind, a process called *free association*. Your dreams may be analyzed to discover hidden conflicts, and your relationships may be explored in detail. The idea is to unlock the subconscious and free you from hidden anger, hurt, frustration, or dependency, any or all of which may have originated in childhood.

Exploratory Psychotherapy

This treatment allows you to open up to the therapist; discuss your problems, issues, and feelings in a supportive environment; and gain some insight into why you do what you do. The therapist may make suggestions or guide you toward certain breakthroughs in self-awareness. Stress relief is a major benefit of this therapy, and stress-related conditions, like asthma and allergies, may improve markedly just by airing problems with a good, sympathetic, and well-trained listener.

Family Therapy

Psychological troubles don't exist in a vacuum; they have a way of reaching out and touching those closest to you. Conversely, if someone in your family is suffering from depression, addiction, anxiety, or stress-related disorders, chances are you'll also feel the effects. Family therapy treats the whole family as a unit (with its complex, interwoven relationships and dynamics) by unraveling family problems and helping the family members become healthier psychologically, both individually and in relation to each other.

FINDING A QUALIFIED PSYCHOTHERAPIST

If you feel like you'd like to talk with a trained professional, by all means do so. But be careful, because lots of people who call themselves counselors have no real training or expertise. For a list of qualified psychotherapists, contact the American Psychological Association's Office of Public Affairs in Washington, D.C. by phone at 202-336-5700, or by E-mail at public.affairs@apa.org.

23

Tried and True Home Remedies

A friend of mine who grew up during the Depression was telling me recently about health care back in the old days. "Back in the thirties," she said, "we didn't go to the doctor until we were practically dying. We just used our home remedies and expected to get well. And you know what? They usually worked!"

My point in telling you this is not to inspire you to give your inhaler the heave-ho or ignore any of the medicines your doctor says you should be taking. Rather, I want to issue a gentle reminder that people have successfully used home remedies—concoctions and little tricks they've whipped up right in their own kitchens—to help ease allergy and asthma symptoms since long before modern medicines were invented. And some of them work just fine, for some people. So, it may be worth your while to take a glance through the home remedies listed in this chapter to see if anything strikes a chord within you. Then, if you feel like experimenting with some of them, go ahead and have fun! But be sure to continue with your regular medication, keep your physician informed of everything you're trying, watch out for reactions, and go easy on the doses.

HOME REMEDIES FOR ALLERGIC RHINITIS OR ASTHMA

When congestion, a runny nose, watery eyes, itching, shortness of breath, or wheezing are driving you crazy, or to prevent them from occurring in the first place, try one or more of the following.

To Prevent Asthma or Allergic Rhinitis

- Drink equal parts of aloe vera juice and wheat grass juice during the spring and fall.
- Drink rose hip tea combined with 1 teaspoon dried, grated grapefruit peel and 1 tablespoon honey, 2 to 3 times a day.
- Eat ½ onion (raw or cooked), daily.
- Make a potion of 1 teaspoon honey plus 5 drops of anise oil, and take before every meal.
- Mix 1 teaspoon of raw, minced garlic with 1 teaspoon vinegar and 1 teaspoon honey. Heat, and take before breakfast each morning.
- Take 1 capsule of black cumin, 3 times daily. Increase to 2 capsules, 3 times a day during pollen season.
- Thinly slice onions and spread them with honey. Cover with plastic wrap and allow to sit overnight, unrefrigerated. Whip in a blender, and take 1 teaspoon before each meal and before bedtime. Refrigerate after blending.
- To prevent asthma, wear a gauze mask when exercising in cold air. This will warm up the air a little before it enters your lungs.
- To prevent pollen allergy, take 1 teaspoon honey made from mixed flowers, daily. Or take 1 tablespoon locally grown honey daily to familiarize your body with local pollens.
- To strengthen the immune system, take 2 tablespoons honey, every day for 4 weeks.

To Ease Shortness of Breath or Wheezing

- Drink strong, caffeinated coffee or strong black tea.

- Hold a clove of garlic between your cheek and your teeth. Don't chew or swallow it; just let the juices flow down your throat.
- Drink a potion of 1 tablespoon whiskey, 1 tablespoon lemon juice, 1 tablespoon honey, and ½ teaspoon grated lemon peel.
- Mix 2 teaspoons cooked, pureed cranberries into 6 ounces of water and drink daily.
- Mix bee pollen and honey to make a thick paste. Smear the paste on the outside of your throat and cover with cheesecloth.
- Slice 1 green apple, pour a cup of boiling water over it, allow to cool, strain, and drink the juice.
- Soak a cloth in castor oil and lay it over your chest for 1 to 2 hours.

To Ease Congestion

- Drink a cup of black cumin tea several times a day.
- Drink at least 8 glasses of water a day.
- When congestion sets in, drink fenugreek tea once every hour, then 4 times daily on subsequent days until congestion clears.
- Each day, eat hot, spicy foods (peppers, curry, mustard, horseradish), or drink a glass of water to which 15 drops of hot pepper sauce have been added.
- Eat chicken soup made with lots of garlic (15 cloves per quart), spiked with curry powder or black pepper.
- Inhale steam from teas made of juniper, pine, eucalyptus, or rosemary.
- Maintain an erect standing or sitting posture.
- Make a mustard plaster from ¼ cup flour and ½ cup dry mustard blended with warm water to form a paste. Apply olive oil to the chest, then spread the mustard mixture between layers of gauze to make a plaster. Lay the plaster on the chest. (Don't apply the paste directly to the skin; it's too irritating.)

- Make natural nose drops from ¼ teaspoon garlic oil, ½ teaspoon salt, ¼ teaspoon powdered vitamin C, and ½ cup warm water. Put a couple of drops in each nostril, hold your head back, and sniff.
- Another nose drop recipe: To 1 quart of water, add 1 tablespoon baking soda and 1 tablespoon pickling salt. Twice a day, using a syringe, squirt some of this mixture into each nostril, while holding your head back. Allow the nose drops to run out of your nose. If you swallow some, don't worry about it; it will just help shrink the inflamed tissues.
- Mix 4 cloves garlic with 1 tablespoon petroleum jelly. Warm slightly, strain, and use as a chest rub.
- Gargle with a glass of water mixed with 20 drops of hot pepper sauce.
- Use a humidifier or vaporizer, adding eucalyptus leaves or apple cider vinegar to the water.
- Drink 1 to 2 glasses of beet, carrot, parsley, spinach, or tomato juice, daily, to counteract the effects of histamine.

HOME REMEDIES FOR ALLERGIC RASHES, DERMATITIS, OR ECZEMA

When you've got a skin reaction, smoothing on an ointment, paste, or cream; applying a compress; or taking a special bath can go a long way toward soothing it, sealing off environmental irritants (however temporarily), and helping it heal. Try one or more of these.

Ointments, Pastes, and Rubs

- Make a paste from powdered goldenseal, vitamin E oil, and honey; apply it to the affected area.
- Mix together baking soda and water to make a paste; apply it to the affected area.

- Several times a day apply calendula ointment, which is made from marigold, an herb with strong anti-inflammatory properties.
- Make a soothing (if messy) paste with crushed charcoal tablets mixed with water.
- Blend powdered slippery elm or mullein leaf with olive oil or wheat germ oil, and smooth over the rash.
- Make a paste of dry slippery elm, 1 teaspoon olive oil, plus a few drops of strained chaparral tea.
- Blend cornstarch mixed with petroleum jelly to make a soothing ointment.
- Make an ointment from powdered turmeric and coconut oil.
- Rub the rash with watermelon rind, then dust with cornstarch.
- Smooth aloe vera gel over the rash.
- Mix together 1 tablespoon vitamin E oil and the contents of 1 vitamin A and 1 vitamin D capsule to make a soothing, healing ointment.
- Wet the rash and gently rub it with an aspirin.

Compresses

- Make a cold compress by stirring ½ cup oatmeal into a quart of simmering water; cook it for 1 to 2 minutes, strain oatmeal, and save the water. Refrigerate this oatmeal water, and, when cold, use it to saturate a clean cloth. Wring out the cloth slightly, fold it, and apply to the affected area.
- Compresses can also be made using cold chaparral tea, warm calendula tea, baking soda, and water, or the refrigerated liquid strained from boiled watercress. Apply compresses frequently.
- Soak a clean cloth in a mixture of 1 quart cold water and 1¼ cups apple cider vinegar. Wrap the cloth around the affected area (e.g., chest, leg, or arm) then add an outer layer

consisting of a dry towel. Leave on the body for 1 to 1½ hours, until treated area is warm.

- Spread plain yogurt on a clean cloth and apply to affected area, securing the cloth with adhesive tape.
- Mix ½ cup apple cider vinegar with ½ cup cold water and 1 teaspoon honey. Dip a piece of gauze into the mixture, lay it over the affected area and fasten with adhesive tape.
- Moisten the rash with the cooled tea of red clover, chickweed, or burdock.
- Plain old petroleum jelly can be applied after using any water-based treatments; if it's carbolated petroleum jelly (available at the drugstore), it may also help ease itching.

Baths

- Take a lukewarm bath to which you've added 1 cup of baking soda. (Don't use hot water; it increases itching.)
- Add 1 quart of strong chamomile tea to a lukewarm bath. (Unless you're allergic to ragweed, chrysanthemums, or other members of the aster and daisy families.)
- Add 1 cup of apple cider vinegar to a lukewarm or cool bath.

FOLK REMEDIES FOR FOOD ALLERGIES

Uh oh! You've got that funny feeling in your stomach that tells you that you've eaten something that's causing a reaction. Quick, try one of these.

To Ease Nausea, Vomiting

- Drink chamomile tea, unless you're allergic to ragweed, chrysanthemums, or other members of the aster and daisy families.

- Drink a mixture of ½ cup warm water, ⅓ cup pear or papaya juice, plus a pinch of cinnamon.
- Drink ginger tea, especially when nausea strikes before breakfast.
- Other teas that may be helpful are peppermint (to soothe) and cascara sagrada (to stimulate the action of the intestines).
- Try a cup of hot water mixed with 1 tablespoon blackstrap molasses.
- Chew alfalfa sprouts, raw potato, or raw celery for a minute or so to ease stomach distress.
- To prevent nausea, drink a mixture of 8 ounces water, 2 tablespoons apple cider vinegar, and 1 tablespoon honey before meals. If diarrhea is present, skip the honey, and substitute mineral water for the plain water.

To Help Prevent Food Allergies

To gain a bit of insurance against allergic reactions to food, consider these:

- Take 2 tablespoons bee pollen every day. (See Chapter 13 for information and cautions regarding bee pollen.)
- Eat yogurt or take 2 acidophilus tablets with every meal.

HOME REMEDIES *CAN* HELP

You can skip the home remedies if you want, but I've found some to be surprisingly effective (e.g., a yogurt compress on a rash). Actually, maybe it isn't all that surprising. Some of these home cures have been in existence for centuries precisely because they do work, at least to some degree.

24

Color Me Healthy with Color Therapy

Color therapy, a long-standing alternative healing system, is based on the premise that color can have a profound influence on the human body. The theory holds that everything in the universe has its own characteristic vibration, including the organs of the body, which vibrate at certain frequencies when they are healthy. Our vibrational patterns become upset when the body is subjected to stresses and strains, whether they're mechanical, environmental, chemical, or otherwise. When this happens, the cells and organs begin to vibrate either faster or slower than they should, and as a result, we become ill. The cure then, according to color therapists, lies in resetting the body's vibrations through color, which itself is pure vibration.

Another tenet of color therapy is that bacteria, viruses, fungi, and cancers all give off light of particular wavelengths. But these invaders are only believed to be dangerous once the body has become strained and some part of it is already vibrating at the wrong frequency. A healthy body, with all parts vibrating properly, should be able to resist disease. It's the unhealthy one, with distorted vibrational patterns, that's in trouble. Allergies, so the theory goes, are just the unpleasant reaction of the body to its disturbed vibrations.

JACK'S EXCELLENT COLOR ADVENTURE

I visited a color therapist, taking along my long-suffering husband, Jack, who's the ultimate skeptic as far as alternative medicine goes. I figured that if color therapy worked for him, there was probably something to it.

Susan, the color therapist, carefully inspected Jack from top to bottom, paying particular attention to the color and condition of his tongue, skin, eyes, and nails. She also asked him about the colors of his urine and stool (which elicited some rolling of his eyes in my direction), as well as the colors of the clothes he usually wears. She listened carefully to his voice, observed the way he carried himself, and checked his pulse. Jack had to describe how he felt physically, mentally, and emotionally as certain colors were mentioned or when Susan held up colored objects. These and other questions helped her zero in on what she called "the color deficiency."

Finally, Susan used a special camera to photograph his aura. A healthy aura, she told us, photographs bright and clear, with colors moving away from the body in waves. But dull colors, dark patches, extra yellow, or other imbalances indicate disease.

In fact, Jack did have some dark patches and some extra yellow in his aura that "proved" that something about his health was not up to snuff. To restore his body to the right vibrational frequency, Susan felt that Jack needed more orange, green, and indigo, colors that are believed to be especially helpful to people with asthma and certain allergies. Medicinal colors are applied through the application of colored light; by ingesting appropriately colored foods or liquids; or by wearing colored threads, clothes, jewelry, and gems. The patient can also meditate on certain colors, colored glass, or gems and can engage in "color breathing." In some cases the color is applied to specific parts of the body in order to strengthen a particular organ.

In general, here's what Jack's colors were supposed to do for him.

Orange

Orange is the color of fire and power. Its apparent effects on the physical body include strengthening the lungs, stimulating the thyroid gland, improving blood circulation, increasing the absorption of nutrients, and relaxing the muscles. Orange releases energy that is used by the spleen and pancreas chakras (energy tunnels that run through the body) and stimulates a profound sense of well-being. Orange foods include carrots, pumpkins, and rutabagas, plus fruits and vegetables with orange skins.

Green

Green builds body tissue. It's also a disinfectant and helps keep blood pressure under control. An emotional stabilizer, green cools and soothes both mind and body. Green foods include any green-colored fruits or vegetables.

Indigo

Indigo helps purify the blood, stimulate the parathyroid, and control bleeding. This color controls the chakra that sits in the middle of the forehead and has a profound influence on vision, healing, and the sense of smell. It's a powerful psychic color, able to raise the vibrational frequency of consciousness to such a point that one may become totally enveloped in the mind and lose track of the body (at least, for a time). Indigo foods include blueberries, blue-skinned fruits and vegetables, grapes, and plums.

TAKING IN THE COLOR

Next we moved on to treatment—which I thought was a real kick! (I participated in the session with Jack because he refused to do it alone.) We were taken to a small, windowless room that was completely cream-colored—including the carpet, textured wallpaper, and even the hardware on the door. Susan brought out bright orange pillows for us to sit on and draped us in soft cashmere shawls—his was a brilliant shade of kelly green, and mine was deepest blue. Susan then used a special projector to fill the room with orange light that radiated softly off the walls and carpet. We were supposed to relax and just "take in" the color. Later she changed the projected color to green, then to dark blue, and finally to yellow, which was supposed to stimulate and cleanse our blood, alimentary canals, and bodies in general.

Afterward, Susan turned the colored lights off, and the room returned to its original cream. We then meditated on one color at a time—we could look at each other's shawls or various colored gems that Susan provided. We also did some color breathing, during which we were supposed to breathe rhythmically, twelve to eighteen times per minute, as we imagined that our bodies were being enveloped in a white light. After about two minutes, we were supposed to focus on a prescribed color or colors as we continued to breathe rhythmically. If you're breathing red, yellow, or orange, Susan told us, you should see it coming up from the earth, through the soles of your feet and into the appropriate body organs. Blue, indigo, and violet, however, is seen as coming down from above into your body, while green is visualized as entering through your navel. We were to continue the rhythmic breathing as we imagined ourselves being bathed in the prescribed color, then return to focusing on white for the final two minutes. (After all that breathing, I was so hyperventilated that I think I saw all the colors of the rainbow!)

While orange, green, and indigo are often selected for asthma and other allergies, yellow (applied to the abdomen) and blue (applied to the face and chest) may be recommended for hay fever. Green, lemon, orange, gold, and turquoise are among the colors that may be chosen for skin problems related to allergies.

JACK'S SUMMATION

Although Jack began his session thinking that color therapy was just plain silly, he was intrigued to find that the color orange was supposed to be good for him. It seems that when he was a child and going through the worst of his asthma, orange was his favorite color. He drank a lot of orange soda and spent a lot of time playing with a certain orange truck. He swears it made him feel better! But, I'm sorry to say, Jack hasn't followed through with his color therapy prescription—he never did any of it again. Still, I know he did enjoy the session and found it relaxing.

FINDING A QUALIFIED COLOR THERAPIST

Few therapists base their practices solely on color therapy, so it may be hard to look one up in the phone book. Usually, it's done as a part of psychotherapy. To find a psychotherapist who also does color therapy, contact the National Register of Health Service Providers in Psychology at 1120 G Street NW, #330, Washington, D.C. 20005; phone 202-783-7663; or visit their website, nationalregister.com.

25

Water Therapy Is *Not* All Wet!

Aaah—cool, clear, delicious water! What could possibly be more refreshing, stimulating, or vital to our being than that wonderful liquid? I remember playing hide and seek outside with my friends for hours when I was a kid. Then suddenly—as if driven by a demon—I'd race into my mother's kitchen, grab a glass, fill it with tap water and chugalug the whole thing at once, making plenty of slurping noises in the process. The fact is, I *was* driven by a demon, my own thirst, which insisted that I drink up once my body's water supply got too low. And it's a good thing, because the majority of the human body (60 percent to be exact) is made up of water. We lose about ten cups of fluid per day through sweating, exhalation, and elimination, so replenishing our water supply throughout the day is absolutely necessary.

Water is a fundamental part of our bodies; it literally makes a life-and-death difference. We can go without food for as long as fifty days, but we can only last a few days without this precious liquid. But besides just keeping us alive, water can bolster and maintain our health by acting as a tonic, diuretic, eliminative, stimulant, sedative, or agent that can reduce fever and pain, induce perspiration, raise body temperature, or ease spasms. And mankind has been well aware of this for hundreds of years (remember the Romans and their special healing baths?). So, the healing art of water therapy, sometimes referred to as *hydrotherapy*, is really nothing new.

WHAT WATER CAN DO FOR YOU

Water therapy is based on the idea that the human body has a physiological response to water that's either ingested or applied to its exterior. This healing art uses good old H_2O as a hot, cold, or lukewarm liquid; steam; or ice, to prompt cleansing and detoxification, ease pain, and change the body's energies in beneficial ways by adding energy to the system and clearing up blockages in energy flow.

Besides all that, water has the ability to:

- Strengthen the body's resistance to disease
- Restore normal body temperature
- Reestablish proper circulation
- Speed the healing of burns
- Detoxify the body and treat several chronic ailments by inducing perspiration
- Relieve constipation
- Flush toxins from the body
- Relieve cramps
- Act as a sedative
- Energize or soothe the nervous system

Water can even serve as a diuretic by helping the kidneys eliminate excess fluid from the body, thus restoring normal fluid balance.

Of course, just any old water won't necessarily do all of these things. In order to be effective, the water must be in the right form. Cold water, for example, restores and energizes the body, and thus increases resistance to disease. Ice or ice water serves as an anesthetic to numb pain or throbbing nerves. Warm water relaxes and sedates, while hot water soothes and quiets the body. Steam has a very different action, helping to draw out toxins via perspiration. Steam is also helpful for loosening up congestion in the chest, while moist, cool air from a humidifier can help relieve problems caused by airborne allergies.

Application and inhalation of water in its various forms aren't the only therapeutic uses of this health-promoting liquid. Just drinking it can bring about many positive effects, like detoxifying and purifying bodily cells, washing away toxins, stimulating the liver and kidneys, diluting body fluids, and increasing the flow of blood.

WATER THERAPY FOR ALLERGIES

There is no single instruction manual for water therapy, so different therapists have somewhat different approaches. These techniques might provide relief from allergies.

- Taking a cool-to-lukewarm bath, to which 1 cup of baking soda has been added, may ease the itching of skin allergies.
- Seawater may help cleanse and tone the skin and bring about relaxation.
- Floating in a sensory deprivation tank is deeply relaxing and relieves stress, thereby soothing allergic reactions.
- Immersion in mineral water helps increase the production of endorphins, which aid in easing pain and inflammation.
- Mild eczema may be soothed by taking a lukewarm bath to which 1 pound of table salt, mineral salt, or Dead Sea salts have been dissolved. (Don't do this if your skin is cracked or you have open sores.)
- Itching caused by rashes or hives may be relieved if the afflicted area is treated with an ice pack or immersed in ice water for a few minutes.

• Hay fever symptoms may subside in response to drinking lots and lots of water (2 and 3 quarts per day). This is considered especially effective if 1 tablespoon of apple cider vinegar and 1 tablespoon of honey are mixed into each cup of water.

• Here's another hay fever remedy. Apply cold compresses to the abdomen every 3 hours throughout the day to tone digestive organs. Immerse your legs and feet in a hot bath. Alternate hot and cold footbaths.

• For congestion, try alternating 20-minute hot showers with 5-minute cold showers. Use the massage or percussive setting on your showerhead, if you have one that offers these options. Direct the spray to your sternum and kidney areas.

• Another congestion remedy is alternating hot and cold footbaths. This sedates and stimulates the body and diverts congestion away from the chest.

• A steam vaporizer can also help ease congestion.

WATER THERAPY FOR ASTHMA

Here's what some hydrotherapists might include in their treatment of asthma (in between attacks), with the aim of strengthening the body and reducing the risk of future attacks:

- Detoxify the body with a hot enema (if constipation is a problem).
- Bathe in cold water up to the feet, calves, or thighs to strengthen the body.
- Drink hot water mixed with lemon juice, honey, or some other cleanser or energizer, daily.
- Apply warm water to the stomach, chest, lower and upper back, and the sides of the rib cage.

And these techniques might be recommended during an asthma attack:

- Take a hot footbath.
- Apply a hot, moist compress to the chest. (Vinegar may be added to the compress.)
- Bathe both hands in hot water.
- Hold an ice compress to the back of the head.
- Inhale steam. You can do this in a steam room or by covering your head with a towel and holding it over a pot of just-boiled water. Eucalyptus leaves may be added to the pot. The steam of sulfur water is also thought to be particularly effective in easing asthma, bronchitis, and sinusitis.

FINDING A QUALIFIED HYDROTHERAPIST

You may be able to find out all you need to know about hydrotherapy by reading a book. (Try *The Complete Book of Water Healing* by the late Dian Dincin Buchman, Ph.D.) But if you'd like the guidance and advice of an expert, contact the American Association of Naturopathic Physicians at 601 Valley Street, Suite 105, Seattle, Washington 98109; phone 206-298-0126; or visit their website, naturopathic.org.

Afterword

Because I don't have allergies or asthma, I can't tell you what's worked best for me. But, as you know, my dear Jack has asthma and allergic rhinitis, and he has served as my occasionally patient guinea pig as I researched the remedies in this book. Here's what brought him the best results:

REDUCE TOXINS IN THE ENVIRONMENT AND CONDITION THE AIR

We bundled up our pillows, mattresses, and box springs in dust mite–proof covers, vacuumed up a storm, and bought a HEPA air filter. We also fixed drippy faucets and wiped down the shower after every use and even fixed the fan above our stove so it would suck up smoke, gas, and cooking odors. We think it's helped—Jack's had a lot less sniffling and sneezing since.

DRINK AN INFUSION OF ELDER FLOWER, YARROW, AND MINT

This has really helped ease his asthmatic cough as well as his hay fever symptoms. He usually starts with the tea as soon as he notices the least little symptom.

REDUCE STRESS

Jack has done this in a couple of different ways. Believe it or not, he's taken up yoga, takes a brisk walk once a day, gets a massage once a month, and has even learned to meditate. His asthma and allergy symptoms really have calmed down quite a bit, and we think at least a part of that is because of these stress relievers.

TRY HYDROTHERAPY

Jack swears by the twenty-minute hot shower followed by a five-minute cold shower that he takes every morning to clear congestion and strengthen his body. He also drinks ten glasses of water per day, saying it helps flush out toxins and keeps him from getting stuffed up.

USE A VAPORIZER

When congestion threatens to keep sleep at bay (his sleep and mine!), we trot out the good old vaporizer, add a few drops of eucalyptus oil to the water, and let it run all night in our bedroom. It's helped.

DRINK ALOE VERA AND WHEAT GRASS JUICE

Here's a short anecdote for you: About four months ago, Jack started drinking a fifty-fifty mixture of these juices every morning to help prevent attacks of allergic rhinitis. He's actually done quiet well since then, but it could be because of the other things I've already mentioned. But the other morning we took a long walk along the border of a golf course that was in the process of being mowed. Freshly cut grass has always made him get stuffy almost instantly, but this time Jack didn't sniff or wheeze once! Jack's theory: the wheat grass juice is helping his system get over his grass allergy, and the aloe juice soothes his mucous membranes. Who am I to argue?

YOU *CAN* DO SOMETHING ABOUT YOUR ASTHMA AND ALLERGIES

Asthma and allergies are whole body conditions that affect you not only physically, but also emotionally, mentally, and spiritually. It only makes sense that they need to be treated on all of these levels. Although Western medicines may be vitally important to controlling your condition, don't just mask your symptoms and ignore the very things that either trigger your illness or make it worse—stress, environmental toxins, food additives, weak breathing apparatus, or poor general health. Clean up your environment, body, nutrition, exercise habits, and your way of thinking. Then try some of these natural remedies that work *with* your body—not against it—to blaze a trail to radiant physical, mental, and emotional health. It's within your grasp—you've just got to reach a little!

Index